Diabetic Diet Cookbook

Healthy Desserts Recipes

Donald R. Butler

Contents

Chapter One

INTRODUCTION

INTRODUCTION

This book will assist you in changing your lifestyle, improving both your physical and mental health while providing you with consistent energy throughout the day.

The low carb diet has been shown in numerous studies to be extremely effective in weight loss. In addition to weight loss, the low carb diet has other health benefits, such as lowering high blood pressure, cholesterol, cardiovascular disease risk, diabetes reversal, and even cancer prevention.

You'll learn how to get the most out of a diabetic diet while still enjoying desserts and sweets. Sweets improve mood by increasing serotonin levels in the body, which is the happy hormone. Many people enjoy sweets, but some are hesitant to consume them due to the added calories, the risk of blood sugar spikes, or other factors. Many people are unaware that there are sugar-free and sugar-free desserts available. It is critical to select sweets that are healthy. You'll find details on which sweeteners are beneficial and which should be avoided inside.

Everybody is affected by sugar cravings.

Sugar cravings can be caused by a variety of factors.

1. You don't eat enough healthy foods or you eat the wrong foods: When you don't eat enough, your body looks for energy elsewhere. Sugar-rich foods, on the other hand, provide instant energy, so you consume them.

2. Bad habits: You develop bad habits as a result of your life experiences. You enjoy eating ice cream or candy bars on a daily basis, for example. Sugar addiction develops from this habit.

3. You eat an unbalanced diet: You will crave sugar if you eat too much starch and not enough protein or fat. Because the calories in a starch-rich dish are quickly absorbed, you won't feel satisfied for long and will crave sugar.

4. You consume excessive amounts of salty foods: Consuming excessive amounts of salt causes sugar cravings.

I propose that we discuss the topic of sweets as a group and use this book to create desserts for any taste or occasion.

Chapter Two

In a diabetic diet, sweeteners are allowed.

In a diabetic diet, sweeteners are allowed.

Here are a few natural low-carb sweeteners that are a good substitute for sugar on a low-carb diet.

• Stevia: Also known as sugar leaf, stevia is a herb. It's a common low-carb dessert substitute. Stevia, a diabetic sweetener that comes in liquid and powder form, is widely used.

• Erythritol: A healthy sugar substitute found in vegetables, fruits, and fermented foods, erythritol is used in low-carb cooking. It's in sugar-free chewing gum, cookies, jam, and ice cream, among other things.

• Monk Fruit: A traditional Chinese fruit, monk fruit is a tasty treat. It contains mogrosides, a 300-fold sweeter compound than sugar. Monk fruit sweeteners are made from these mogrosides, which are extracted from the fruit. There are no calories or carbs in monk fruit sweeteners.

• Xylitol: Xylitol is a sugar alcohol found in the fiber of some fruits and vegetables. Tea, coffee, shakes, and smoothies all contain xylitol as a flavoring. Xylitol aids in the prevention of osteoporosis and is beneficial to dental health.

Swerve is a zero-calorie sweetener that is made naturally. Swerve is an erythritol-based sweetener. Swerve dissolves completely, making it a great option for drinks and teas.

Low-Carb Sweeteners Have These Advantages:

• Stevia aids in the reduction of blood sugar. Stevia extracts helped type-2 diabetes patients reduce their post-meal sugar by 16 to 18 percent, according to one study. • Erythritol is a popular sweetener due to its low calorie content, which makes it a good choice for weight loss. In type-2 diabetics, erythritol aids in the improvement of blood vessel function.

• Monk fruits can help you lose weight. It's a calorie-free sweetener that can help people lose weight by lowering their total calorie intake. Because of its anti-infection properties, monk fruit aids in limiting the growth of bacteria. It's good for bacteria in the mouth that can lead to tooth decay.

• Xylitol helps to strengthen your bones by remineralizing bone tissue. Middle ear infections can be reduced with xylitol. Chewing gum or syrup are used to deliver it.

• Swerve is primarily used in baking because it caramelizes and browns in the same way that sugar does.

sugar as it is Swerve is a zero-calorie, non-glycemic sweetener that is safe for diabetics because it has no effect on blood sugar levels.

Sweeteners Can Be Harmful:

• Sucralose should be used with caution because high doses can cause harmful side effects. • Maltitol isn't a good option because 40% of the sweetener is absorbed in the small intestine, causing blood sugar levels to rise, especially in diabetics.

• Fructose is directly absorbed by the liver, causing fatty liver, central obesity, and insulin resistance. Over time, fructose causes a great deal of metabolic harm.

Avoid the following sweeteners:

Here are a few sweeteners to stay away from when you're on a diabetic diet. These sweeteners are high in carbohydrates, which causes blood sugar levels to rise.

• Maple Syrup: Although maple syrup is high in micronutrients such as zinc and manganese, it is also high in sugar and carbs, making it unsuitable for a low-carb diet.

• Honey: Honey is a great alternative to refined sugar because it is rich in nutrients and antioxidants. It is, however, still high in carbs and calories, making it unsuitable for a diabetic diet.

• Agave nectar is high in fructose, which lowers insulin sensitivity. It is not suitable for a diabetic diet because it makes it difficult for your body to regulate blood sugar levels.

• Coconut sugar: Coconut sugar has a higher fructose content than regular sugar and is absorbed more slowly.

• Dates: Dates are a natural sweetener that can be added to a variety of desserts. It is high in carbohydrates and contains vitamins, minerals, and a small amount of fiber.

• Maltodextrin: Maltodextrin is a type of sweetener made from a starchy plant, such as wheat or corn, and it has the same carbohydrate and calorie content as regular sugar.

Chapter Three

Diabetic Diet's Advantages

This chapter will conclude with a discussion of the Diabetic Diet's Advantages.

It aids in the prevention and management of diabetes in the following ways: Blood sugar levels rise when you eat a carb-heavy diet. The release of insulin is triggered by an increase in blood sugar levels, and your cells eventually become insulin resistant, leading to diabetes. You drastically reduce your carb and sugar intake when you follow a low carb diet. They both cause a spike in blood sugar. Your body doesn't need to release insulin to manage blood sugar levels when there isn't much. As a result, you can either prevent diabetes from developing or manage it if you already have it.

2. It curbs your appetite: The diabetic diet curbs your desire for sugary, carbohydrate-laden junk food.

3. The diabetic diet aids in the reduction of dangerous abdominal fat, which can lead to a variety of chronic diseases, including diabetes. The low carb diet helps you lose body fat and lower your risk of disease by utilizing stored body fat and fat you consume as energy.

4. The diabetic diet lowers triglyceride levels in the blood: High triglyceride levels in the blood can increase your risk of diabetes and heart disease. Triglyceride levels are lower when you follow a low-carb diet.

5. A diabetic diet improves mental focus: Unhealthy carbohydrate-rich diets cause brain fog or a lack of mental focus. Low-carb eating improves mental focus and productivity.

Chapter Four

Low-Carb Diet

Baking Suggestions for a Low-Carb Diet

1. Almond flour and almond meal are not the same: They are both made from almonds but not the same. Almond flour is made from blanched almonds without their skins. Almond meal is made with almonds with the skin. The fineness of almond flour makes it interchangeable with flour, but the almond meal is not.

2. Using low-carb flours: You can use low carb flours such as almond or coconut flour for baking, but you have to stick to recipes that are created for low-carb baking. You can't interchange all-purpose flour with almond flour or coconut flour.

3. Choose ingredients wisely: For example, if your recipe calls for flax meal, then use golden flax meal. Seasoned bakers recommend golden flax meal because it is less gummy compared to standard flax meal.

4. Use room temperature butter and cream cheese: Use room temperature dairy products, so they blend well. Take out your eggs, buttercream cheese, and other refrigerated ingredients 30 minutes before baking. Unless it is otherwise specified, use room temperature eggs and liquids.

5. Using dairy: Avoid milk and use heavy cream because it is low in carb. If the recipe needs more liquid, then add water or use unsweetened almond or coconut milk.

6. Using baking powder or soda: Compared to normal baking, low-carb baking needs more baking powder or soda to keep them light. The low-carb flour alternatives, such as coconut or almond flour, are a bit denser compared to regular flour. So you need a bit more leavening agent compared to regular recipes.

7. Grease your pans well: Compared to traditional recipes, low-carb batters tend to be a bit stickier. So grease your baking pans well. You may need to use butter to grease the pan and then use parchment paper.

8. Choose only low-carb recipes for low-carb baking: Don't try to convert regular recipes to low carb because they won't work.

9. Experiment when you have experience: Once you baked low-carb goods a few times, start to experiment and develop your own recipes.

10. Use properly softened cream cheese and butter: If your baking ingredients are too cold, they won't get evenly distributed and result in uneven baking.

11. Don't pack unless mentioned: When measuring low-carb flours, don't pack unless specified.

12. Use unsalted butter: Use unsalted butter unless mentioned otherwise.

13. Use large eggs.

14. Oven and stovetop temperatures vary: So start to check on your baked product before

the finished time.

15. Melting the chocolate: Use a double boiler to melt your chocolate because chocolate melts smoothly with a gentle heat.

16. Cool properly then cut: Low-carb items continue to firm up as they cool. So cool your baked goods then slice.

Chapter Five

CAKE RECIPES

CAKE RECIPES\sChocolate Coffee Cake

Prep time: 20 minutes Cook time: 1 hour Servings: 6

• 6 eggs\s• ½ cup butter, melted\s• 1/3 cup plus 1 tbsp. almond flour\s• 1/3 cup cacao powder

• 3 oz unsweetened chocolate, melted\s• ½ cup stevia\s• ½ cup Erythritol\s• 2 tbsp vanilla extract\s• ½ tsp salt\s• ½ tsp baking soda\s• 1 tsp ground cinnamon\s• ½ tsp cayenne pepper

1. Preheat the oven to 325F. Line a loaf pan with wax paper. Grease wax paper with butter.

2. Into a small bowl, add cayenne, cinnamon, almond flour, sifted cocoa, salt, and baking soda.

3. In a food processor, combine vanilla, stevia, Erythritol, and eggs. Pulse a few times to beat together. Add melted butter and chocolate and process for 1 minute.

4. Add the dry ingredients to the food processor and pulse to combine.

5. Pour batter into the pan. Bake until your desired doneness is reached, about 1 hour. Check after 55 minutes with a toothpick.

6. Let cool completely in the pan. Remove from pan and serve.

• Calories: 314

• Fat: 32.4g • Carbs: 6.2g • Protein: 11.7g

Chapter Six

Raspberry Lemon Cake

Raspberry Lemon Cake

Prep time: 15 minutes Cook time: 30 minutes Servings: 8

• 2 tbsp butter, cut into 4 pieces (and more if needed) • 4 eggs • 4 ounces cream cheese • ¼ cup coconut flour • ¼ cup Erythritol • 1 ½ tsp baking powder

• 1 tsp vanilla extract • 1 tbsp lemon zest • ¼ cup raspberries • Nonstick cooking spray For Frosting

• 1 tbsp heavy cream • ½ tsp vanilla • 2 tsp fresh lemon juice • 3 tbsp swerve • 4 oz cream cheese, softened

1. Preheat the oven to 425F. Coat a baking pan with cooking spray.

2. Put the four pieces of butter in the baking pan.

3. Place the pan in the oven for about 2 to 3 minutes to melt the butter, but do not brown. Remove from the oven.

4. In a blender, process the eggs, cream cheese, coconut flour, erythritol, baking powder, vanilla, and lemon zest until mixed.

5. Pour the batter into the baking pan with melted butter.

6. Drop the raspberries into the cake.

7. Bake for 15 minutes.

8. Meanwhile, make the frosting. In a large bowl add all the frosting ingredients: heavy cream, vanilla, lemon juice, swerve, and cream cheese and beat using a hand mixer until creamy.

9. Once the cake is cool completely then frost cake using prepared cream.

• Calories: 146

• Fat: 11g • Carbs: 5g • Protein: 5.4g

Prep time: 10 minutes Cook time: 20 minutes Servings: 8

• Nonstick cooking spray

• 2 tbsp butter, cut into 4 pieces, plus more if needed • 4 eggs • 4 ounces cream cheese • ¼ cup coconut flour • ¼ cup Erythritol • 1 ½ tsp baking powder • 1 tsp vanilla extract • 1 tbsp lemon zest • ¼ cup blueberries

1. Preheat the oven to 425F. Coat a baking pan with cooking spray.

2. Put the four pieces of butter in the baking pan.

3. Place the pan in the oven for about 2 to 3 minutes to melt the butter, but do not brown. Remove from the oven.

4. In a blender, process the eggs, cream cheese, coconut flour, Erythritol, baking powder, vanilla, and lemon zest until mixed.

5. Pour the batter into the baking pan with melted butter.

6. Drop the blueberries into the cake.

7. Bake for 15 minutes and serve.

• Calories: 174

• Fat: 14g • Carbs: 4g • Protein: 5.1g

Prep time: 15 minutes

Cook time: 2 hours 50 minutes

Servings: 12 slices

Ingredients For the filling

• 2 3/4 cup almond flour • 1 ½ cups sweetener, granulated • 2 tsp baking powder, gluten-free • ½ cup butter, melted • 4 oz dark chocolate, stevia sweetened • ½ cup cocoa powder, unsweetened • 6 large eggs • 1 avocado, pureed • 2 tsp vanilla extract, sugar-free • 1 tsp salt For the icing • 1/2 cup butter

• Liquid stevia, to taste • 1/2 cup cocoa powder, unsweetened • 1/8 tsp. salt

Instructions

Make the cake:

1. Set your stove to the temperature of 350° F. Use cooking spray or heavily butter an 8- inch cake pan or cover with parchment lining.

2. In a regular dish, combine the eggs, avocado, baking powder, and vanilla extract until mixed well.

3. Add the almond flour, sweetener, dark chocolate and butter until incorporated. Then add the salt and cacao powder until smooth.

4. Distribute the cake batter into the prepped pan and heat in the stove for 45 minutes. Using a wooden stick, press it into the middle of the cake to make sure it is baked properly.

5. Transfer to the counter and remove from the pan. Set to the side. Make the frosting:

1. Heat a saucepan to liquefy the butter completely.

2. Combine the cacao powder, salt, and liquid stevia and mix until smooth.

3. Let the icing completely cool before frosting the cake.

4. Remember to frost the middle first. Then to complete the frosting, down the sides.

Nutrition Facts (Per Serving)

• Calories: 205

• Fat: 18g • Carbs: 2.2g • Protein: 6g

Prep time: 10 minutes Cook time: 20 minutes Servings: 12

• 9 ounces almond meal • 6 eggs • 2 peaches, stoned, cut into quarters • 1 tsp vanilla extract • 1 tsp baking powder • 4 tbsp Swerve

• A pinch of salt • 2 tbsp orange zest • 2 ounces stevia • 4 ounces cream cheese • 4 ounces plain Greek yogurt

1. Chop the peaches in a food processor.

2. Put to the peaches Swerve, almond meal, eggs, baking powder, vanilla extract, a pinch of salt. Pulse well. Divide the dough into two baking tins.

3. Place in an oven at 350F. Bake for 20 minutes.

4. In a separate bowl, mix cream cheese, yogurt, orange zest, stevia, and stir well.

5. Place the first crust on a plate. Add half of the cream cheese mixture. Add the other cake layer.

6. Top with the remaining cream cheese mixture.

7. Spread it well. Slice and serve.

• Calories: 206

• Fat: 16.5g • Carbs: 5.1g • Protein: 8.7g

Prep time: 20 minutes Cook time: 30 minutes Servings: 12 • ½ cup butter, softened • 4 large lemons, chopped • ¼ cup sugar-free maple syrup • ½ cup Erythritol • 1 tsp vanilla extract • ½ cup almond flour • 3 large eggs, lightly beaten • ½ cup heavy cream • 1 tbsp swerve confectioner's sugar

1. Throw the lemons in a saucepan. Add in sugar-free maple syrup and simmer over low heat for 10 minutes. Pour the mixture into a blender and process until smooth. Pour into a jar and set aside.

2. Preheat oven to 350 F. Grease two (8-inch) springform pans with cooking spray and line with parchment paper.

3. In a bowl, cream the butter, erythritol, and vanilla extract with an electric whisk until light and fluffy. Pour in the eggs gradually while beating until fully mixed. Carefully fold in the almond flour and share the mixture into the cake pans.

4. Bake for 30 minutes or until springy when touched and a toothpick inserted comes out clean.

5. Remove and let cool for 5 minutes before turning out onto a wire rack.

6. In a bowl, whip heavy cream until a soft peak forms. Spoon onto the bottom sides of the cake and spread the lemon puree on top. Sandwich both cakes and sift confectioner's sugar on top.

7. Slice and serve.

• Calories: 270

• Fat: 24g • Carb: 4.4g • Protein: 6.1g

Prep time: 20 minutes

Cook time: 1 hour 30 minutes

Servings: 12 slices

Ingredients For the cake • 1 cup Swerve sweetener, granulated • 2 ½ tsp baking powder, gluten-free • ½ cup Sukrin Gold brown sugar substitute • 1 cup butter, unsalted and room temperature

• 2 ½ cups almond flour, finely milled • ½ cup coconut, unsweetened and flaked • 2 cups grated carrots • ½ cup heavy whipping cream • 2 tsp ground ginger • 1 cup pecans, raw and roughly chopped • 5 large eggs • ½ tsp ground nutmeg • 2 tbsp cinnamon powder • ½ tsp salt For the frosting • 3/4 cup heavy whipping cream • 1 ¼ cup Swerve sweetener, confectioner • 3/4 cup unsalted butter, softened • 12 oz cream cheese, full fat For the topping • 1 cup pecans, raw and roughly chopped

Instructions

Make the cake:

1. Set your stove to the temperature of 350° F. Use cooking spray or heavily butter the sides and base of two 9 inch cake pans. Cover them with baking paper.

2. In a regular dish, blend the sweetener and butter until mixed well. Add 1 egg. Beat into the mixture and repeat until all eggs are combined.

3. Stir the heavy whipping cream, brown sugar and carrots into the batter until thoroughly incorporated.

4. In a big dish, whisk the almond flour remove the lumps if present.

5. Then add the cinnamon powder, ground nutmeg, baking powder, and ground ginger.

6. Slowly combine the flour to the cake batter. Incorporate the coconut and pecans until mixed together.

7. Evenly distribute the batter in the prepared cake pans and heat in the stove for 35 minutes. Use a toothpick in the

middle of the cake to make sure it is baked properly.

8. Remove to the counter and let it rest for 10 minutes. Unlock the pan and set the cake to the side until ready to frost.

Make the frosting:

1. Using a food processor on high, whisk the butter, sweetener and cream cheese for 3 minutes. Scrape the dish with a rubber scraper as necessary and continue to blend until fully incorporated.

2. Pour the heavy whipping cream into the frosting and beat for an additional 2 minutes until airy.

3. Move the first layer on a cake platter and apply the frosting to the top, keeping an even layer. Put the second cake above and apply frosting to the top.

4. Then frost the edges of the layers of cake keeping the frosting as even as possible.

5. Dust the top with the chopped pecans, cut into slices and serve.

Tricks and Tips: If you do not want to go through all the trouble of the layered cake, you can always use a 13 x 9 cake pan and add the frosting to keep the cake in a cake pan.

Nutrition Facts (Per Serving)

• Calories: 422

• Fat: 29g • Carbs: 4.9g • Protein: 8g

Prep time: 12 minutes Cook time: 9 minutes Servings: 2 • 2 ounces 85 percent cocoa chocolate • 1 tbsp almond flour • 2 ounces ghee, plus more for greasing • 2 eggs • 1 tsp vanilla extract • 2 tbsp powdered Erythritol • 1 tbsp granulated Erythritol • 1/8 tsp sea salt • 2 tbsp 85 percent chocolate chunks • Fresh raspberries, almond butter for garnish

1. Preheat the oven to 350F.

2. Grease two ramekins with ghee.

3. Melt 2 ounces ghee and chocolate in a saucepan on low heat. Stir to combine and set aside.

4. Whisk eggs, salt, and vanilla until frothy.

5. Add egg mixture, the chocolate mixture, along with sweetener and almond flour. Mix to combine.

6. Fill two ramekins halfway with batter.

7. Add chocolate chunks, and add the remaining batter.

8. Bake until tops are set but still jiggly, about 9 minutes.

9. Cool, garnish, and serve.

• Calories: 484

• Fat: 43g • Carbs: 4.4g • Protein: 9.8g

Prep time: 10 minutes Cook time: 35 minutes Servings: 12

• ¾ cup butter, softened • 1 cup of water • 1 cup liquid Splenda • ½ cup heavy cream • 1 tsp vanilla • 1 ½ cup almond flour • ½ cup coconut flour, sifted • ¼ tsp salt • 2 tsp baking powder

1. In a clean mixing bowl, place all the ingredients. Mix well and beat with a hand mixer until creamy

2. If the batter is too stiff, add a little water.

3. Spread in a greased pan and bake at 350F until golden and firm to the touch. Bake for about 30 to 35 minutes.

4. Cool completely before serving.

• Calories: 216

• Fat: 19.6g • Carbs: 7g • Protein: 4.3g

Prep time: 20 minutes Cook time: 40 minutes Servings: 12
Cake • 2 cups almond flour • ½ cup Swerve sweetener • 2 tbsp unflavored whey protein powder • 2 tsp baking powder • ¼ tsp salt • ½ cup butter, melted • 1 large egg • ½ tsp vanilla extract Filling

• 8 ounces cream cheese, softened • ½ cup butter, softened • ¾ cup powdered Swerve • 2 large eggs • ½ tsp vanilla extract • Powdered Swerve for dusting

1. Preheat the oven to 325°F and lightly grease a 9 x 13 baking pan.

2. In a large bowl, combine the almond flour, sweetener, protein powder, baking powder, and salt. Add the butter, egg, and vanilla extract and stir to combine well. Press into the bottom and partway up the sides of the prepared baking pan.

3. In another large bowl, beat the cream cheese and butter together until smooth. Beat in the sweetener until well combined, then beat in the eggs and vanilla until smooth.

4. Pour the filling over the crust. Bake 35 to 45 minutes, until the filling is mostly set, but the center still jiggles, and the edges are just golden-brown.

5. Remove and let cool, then dust with powdered Swerve and cut into bars.

• Calories: 286

• Fat: 22g • Carb: 3g • Protein: 7g

Cheesecake Pie made with pumpkin

Prep time: 10 minutes Cook time: 1 hour Servings: 8

• 1 tsp. vanilla extract • 1 tsp. cinnamon • ½ tsp. ginger, ground • 3 eggs • 8 oz. cream cheese, softened • 2 cups pumpkin, pureed • ¾ cup sugar-free (keto) sweetener • ½ tsp. salt • ½ tsp. nutmeg, ground • ½ tsp. cloves, ground • 1 recipe Keto pie crust

1. Roll out the dough and spread out on a pie dish. Crimp the edges.

2. Whisk the cream cheese in a separate bowl until fluffy.

3. In another clean bowl combine the spices and sweetener.

4. Spoon the spice seasoning into the cream cheese and mix until fully mixed and fluffy.

5. Add one egg to this bowl and mix well. Do the same with the remaining eggs.

6. Then add the pumpkin and vanilla extract to the mixture. Whip until mixed.

7. Transfer the mixture to the crust in the pie dish. Bake for 40 minutes at 350F.

8. Refrigerate for 30 minutes or so. Serve when set .

• Calories: 284

• Fat: 23g • Carbs: 3g • Protein: 8g

Chapter Seven

New Dessert

Prep time: 15 minutes + Chilling Cook time: 30 minutes

Servings: 4

Piecrust • ¼ cup almond flour + extra for dusting • 3 tbsp coconut flour • ½ tsp salt • ¼ cup butter, cold and crumbled • 3 tbsp Erythritol • 1 ½ tsp vanilla extract • 4 whole eggs Filling • 2 ¼ cup strawberries and blackberries • 1 cup Erythritol + extra for sprinkling • 1 vanilla pod, bean paste extracted • 1 egg, beaten

1. In a large bowl, mix the almond flour, coconut flour, and salt. Add the butter and mix with an electric hand mixer until crumbly. Add the erythritol and vanilla extract until mixed in.

Then, pour in the 4 eggs one after another while mixing until formed into a ball.

2. Flatten the dough a clean flat surface, cover in plastic wrap, and refrigerate for 1 hour.

3. Preheat oven to 350 F and grease a pie pan with cooking spray.

4. Lightly dust a clean flat surface with almond flour, unwrap the dough, and roll out the dough into a large rectangle, ½ - inch thickness and fit into a pie pan. Pour some baking beans onto the pastry and bake in the oven until golden. Remove after, pour pout the baking beans, and allow cooling.

5. Toss the berries with the erythritol and vanilla bean paste in a mixing bowl.

6. Spoon the filling into the pie shell, level with a spoon, and cover the berries with pastry strips to make a lattice top. Bake for 30 minutes, or until the fruit is bubbling and the pie is golden brown, brushing with the beaten egg and sprinkling with more erythritol as needed.

7. Remove from the oven and set aside to cool before slicing and serving with whipped cream.

• There are 184 calories in a single serving of this recipe.

18.8 g fat, 3.3 g carbohydrate, 9.2 g protein

Tart apple

10 minute prep time 55-minute time to cook 8 people

1 tsp cinnamon • 1/3 cup erythritol • 2 cups almond flour • 6 tbsp melted butter for the crust • 14 cup erythritol • 12 tsp. cinnamon • 14 cup butter • 12 tsp. lemon juice • 3 cups peeled, cored, and sliced apples for the filling

1. Preheat oven to 375 degrees Fahrenheit (190 degrees Celsius).

2. To make the crust, combine butter, cinnamon, Swerve, and almond flour in a mixing bowl and stir until crumbly.

3. Press the crust mixture evenly into the bottom of a springform pan.

4. Cook the crust for 5 minutes in the oven.

5. Mix apple slices and lemon juice in a bowl for the filling.

6. In a circular pattern, arrange apple slices on the bottom of the baked crust. After that, lightly press down.

7. Microwave butter, Swerve, and cinnamon for 1 minute in a microwave-safe bowl. Pour over apple slices, whisking until smooth.

8. Preheat the oven to 350°F and bake for 30 minutes. Remove the baked apple slices from the oven and lightly press with a fork.

9. Increase the oven temperature to 350 degrees Fahrenheit and bake for an additional 20 minutes.

10. Take the pan out of the oven and set it aside to cool completely.

11. Serve by cutting into slices.

• 302 kcal

26 g of fat

• 7 g carbs

7 grams of protein

Pie made with chocolate

3 hr. 10 min. prep time 20-minute cook time Number of servings: 10

12 tsp baking powder • 12 cup almond flour • A pinch of salt • 1/3 cup stevia • 1 egg • 12 tsp vanilla extract • 3 tbsp butter Filler

4 tbsp. butter • 1 tbsp. vanilla extract

12 cup stevia • 12 cup cocoa powder • 2 tsp. granulated stevia • 1 cup whipping cream • 1 tsp. vanilla extract

Instructions

1. Preheat oven to 350°F and grease a springform pan with 1 tablespoon butter.

2. Stir baking powder, almond flour, 1/3 cup stevia, and a pinch of salt together in a mixing bowl.

3. Combine 3 tbsp. butter, 1 12 tsp. vanilla extract, and 3 tbsp. flour in a large mixing bowl. To make a dough, combine all of the ingredients in a mixing bowl and stir well.

4. Pour into a springform pan and bake for 11 minutes at 375°F. Preheat the oven to 350°F and remove the pie crust.

5. Finally, use tin foil to cover the dish. Return to the oven for another 8 minutes. Set aside after that.

6. Meanwhile, combine cream cheese, 4 tablespoons butter, sour cream, 1 tablespoon vanilla essence, chocolate powder, and 12 cup stevia in a mixing bowl and well combine.

7. In a separate dish, whisk together whipping cream, 2 teaspoons stevia, and 1 teaspoon vanilla extract.

8. Combine the two contents in a pie shell and bake. Refrigerate for a few hours after spreading.

Serve after three hours.

Facts on Nutrition (Per Serving)

• There are 420 calories in a single serving of this recipe.

• 38 grams of fat; 6 grams of carbohydrates; 8 grams of protein

10 minute prep time 20-minute cook time 4 people

12 cup Swerve • 1 tsp baking powder • 1 cup almond meal • 1 tsp vanilla extract • 5 egg whites • 12 oz strawberries

1 lemon (zested)

1. Preheat oven to 375 degrees Fahrenheit (190 degrees Celsius).

2. To make the egg whites frothy and smooth, whisk them until they are foamy and smooth.

3. Combine all other ingredients, save the strawberries, in a large mixing bowl and well combine.

4. Spray a muffin tin with nonstick cooking spray. Bake for 15-20 minutes, or until the cake is golden brown, in a baking dish with the tart mixture.

5. Place strawberries on top and let aside to cool.

6. Serve.

• There are 361 calories in 361 calories in 361 calories in 361 calories in 361

• 34 grams of fat; 5 grams of carbohydrates; 10 grams of protein

15 minute prep time 15-minute time to cook 8 people

14 cup Swerve • 14 cup melted butter • 2 cups almond flour For the crust • 1 egg • 1 tsp vanilla • 2 tbsp heavy cream, for the filling

• a quarter cup of Swerve • six ounces of mascarpone cheese • a third of a cup of lemon curd

1. Lightly grease a tart pan. Remove the item from circulation.

2. Preheat oven to 350 degrees Fahrenheit (180 degrees Celsius).

3. In a food processor, combine almond flour, vanilla, Swerve, egg, and butter until a dough forms.

4. Press the dough evenly into the tart pan.

5. Using a fork, prick the crust, then top with parchment paper and dry beans.

6. Cook for 15 minutes in the oven.

7. Take the dish out of the oven and set it aside. Allow to cool fully before removing from the oven.

8. In a food processor, blend together the lemon curd, heavy cream, Swerve, and mascarpone until smooth and creamy.

9. Evenly distribute the filling mixture in the cooked crust. Set aside for 2 hours in the fridge.

10. Serve by cutting into slices.

• There are 369 calories in 369 calories in 369 calories in 369 calories in 369

• 24g fat; 6g carbohydrate; 9g protein

10 minute prep time 20-minute cook time For the filling, 6 servings

• 2 Hass avocados • 14 cup lime juice • 2 tablespoons lime zest • 1 tablespoon coconut oil • 14 teaspoon vanilla essence • 14 teaspoon kosher salt • 2 teaspoon Stevia powder Shells for tarts

• 1 egg • 12 tsp salt • 2 tsp Stevia powder • 1 tbsp lime zest • 1/3 cup almond butter • 1 tbsp coconut oil

To make the filling, start by following the steps below:

Mix all of the filling ingredients in a food processor. Blend until the mixture is completely smooth.

2. Place in the refrigerator for an hour before spooning into tart shells.

3. To make the tart shells, mix together all of the wet ingredients. Stir in the lime zest, salt, and stevia until all of the ingredients are well combined.

4. To produce a firm dough, add the flax meal and mix well.

5. Fill six 3" silicone tart shells with the mixture.

6. Cook for 20 minutes at 350°F in the oven.

7. Allow to cool completely before serving, garnished with lime zest and a lemon slice.

• There are 338 calories in 338 calories in 338 calories in 338 calories in 338

• 28g fat; 5g carbohydrate; 9g protein

20-minute prep time 40-minute time to cook 9 people

12 cup coconut flour • 1/3 cup melted butter • 1 egg • 14 teaspoon liquid Stevia for the pie crust 2 12 cup mixed berries • 1/3 cup erythritol • 1 tbsp coconut flour Crumble topping • 12 cup almond flour • 14 cup erythritol • 1 tsp cinnamon powdered • 4 tbsp cold butter, cut in fourths

1. Preheat oven to 375 degrees Fahrenheit (190 degrees Celsius). Coat a pan with cooking spray.

2. Toss all of the fruit filling ingredients together in a mixing basin. Toss the fruit with coconut flour and erythritol to lightly coat it. Remove the item from circulation. Allow 15 minutes for rest.

3. Incorporate all of the pie crust ingredients in a mixing dish and stir to combine.

4. Press the dough evenly into the bottom of the pan to completely cover it. Remove the item from circulation.

5. In a separate dish, using a big fork, mix together all of the crumble topping ingredients.

6. Combine all of the ingredients in a tiny crumbly chunk in the butter.

7. Spoon the fruit mixture over the top of the pie crust in the pan and distribute it evenly.

8. Scatter crumble mixture on top in tiny quantities.

9. Bake for 35 to 40 minutes on the middle rack, until the topping is golden brown.

10. Allow to cool for approximately 20 minutes, or until the fruit mixture has firmed and set.

• 198 kcal

16 g of fat

• 5.6 g carbohydrate • 3.1 g protein

Fruit Galette with Vanilla and Passion

Time to prepare: 10 minutes plus time to cool 30 minute time to cook

Ingredients/Servings: 4

12 cup butter, heated • 1 cup crumbled almond biscuits
Filling

• 1 12 cup mascarpone cheese • 34 cup swerve sugar • 12 cup whipping cream • 1 teaspoon vanilla bean paste • 4-6 tablespoons cold water • 1 tablespoon gelatin powder 14 cup room temperature water • 1 cup passion fruit pulp • 14 cup swerve confectioner's sugar • 1 teaspoon gelatin powder

Instructions

1. Toss broken biscuits with melted butter in a mixing basin. Set aside in the fridge after spooning into a spring-form pan and leveling with the back of a spoon.

2. In a separate bowl, combine the mascarpone cheese, swerve sugar, and vanilla paste; whisk until smooth with a hand mixer; set aside.

3. Combine 2 tbsp cold water and 1 tbsp gelatin powder in a third mixing dish. Allow for a 5-minute dissolving period.

4. Fold the cheese mixture carefully with the gelatin liquid and the whipped cream.

5. Take the spring-form pan out of the freezer and pour the mixture into it. Make your way back to the refrigerator. Then, when you're out of ingredients, pour in the confectioner's sugar and 14 cup of water and continue the dissolving procedure with the remaining gelatin.

6. Add the passion fruit pulp to the mixture and whisk to combine.

7. Take the cake out of the oven and pour the jelly on top. To level the jelly, swirl the pan. Refrigerate the pan for another 2 hours to cool.

Remove and unlock the spring-pan after it has fully set. Remove the cake from the pan and cut it into slices.

Facts on Nutrition (Per Serving)

• There are 315 calories in a single serving of this dish.

28 g fat, 4.8 g carbohydrate, 9.2 g protein

A cheesecake from New York

10 minute prep time 1 hour of cooking 16 portions

12 tsp cinnamon, crushed • 5 tbsp salted butter • 3 tbsp sugar-free (keto) sweetener • 6 oz sliced almonds • 3 eggs to make the filling

• 32 ounces melted cream cheese • 16 ounces sour cream • 34 cup sugar-free (keto) sweetener

In a food processor, grind the almonds. Until you have a fine powder.

2. Add the cinnamon and sweetener.

3. Pulse one more with the butter.

4. Press the butter mixture down into a baking pan. Remove from the equation.

5. Whip the cream cheese till light and fluffy to produce the filling.

6. Whisk in the sweetener until smooth.

7. Combine the eggs, one at a time, into the mixture.

8. Fold in the sour cream and vanilla extract.

9. Spread the cream mixture evenly over the crust.

10. Bake the cheesecake for an hour at 300°F, or until gently browned on top.

11. Remove the pan from the oven and let it there for an hour. After that, chill for at least 24 hours before serving.

• There are 356 calories in a single serving of this recipe.

• 34 g fat • 4 g carbohydrate • 7.2 g protein

Chapter Eight

Delicious Dessert

10 minute prep time

1 hour and 15 minutes to prepare

Ingredients/Servings: 12

Filler

• 1 12 cup sugar equivalent substitute • 5 (8-ounce) packages softened cream cheese

• There are three eggs

• 12 c. yogurt (Greek)

• 1 tblsp lemon juice (optional)

• 12 tsp vanilla extract (optional) Crust

• 2 tbsp sugar equivalent substitute • 1 cup whole almonds, coarsely crushed in a processor

• melted butter (four tablespoons) 1 cup heavy whipping cream, unsweetened • 2 tbsp sugar substitute

Instructions

To make the crust, start with the following steps:

1. In a large mixing bowl, combine the sweetener, butter, and almond meal; press into the bottom of a 10-inch springform pan. Refrigerate.

To make the filling, follow these instructions.

Preheat the oven to 325 degrees Fahrenheit (180 degrees Celsius).

2. In a mixer fitted with a paddle attachment, beat cream cheese and sweetener for one minute on medium speed.

3. Blend in the eggs one at a time on low speed until thoroughly combined.

4. Combine the lemon juice, Greek yogurt, and vanilla extract in a mixing bowl and whisk until smooth.

5. Fill the crust with the mixture.

6. Place a pan of water in the rack beneath the cheesecake.

7. Bake for 1 hour 15 minutes to 90 minutes, or until the pudding is set.

8. Set aside for 15 minutes to cool on a cooling rack.

9. Refrigerate for a few hours.

10. Unsweetened cream, fruits, or berries can be used to decorate ready-made cheesecake.

Facts on Nutrition (Per Serving)

• There are 368 calories in 368 calories in 368 calories in 368 calories in 368

• 43g fat; 4.9g carbohydrates; 11g protein

10 minute prep time 20-minute cook time 9 people

• 12 tsp. baking powder • 4 tbsp. Swerve • 5 ounces melted coconut oil

• 12 cup blueberries • 1 teaspoon vanilla extract • 4 ounces cream cheese

1. In a mixing bowl, whisk together the coconut oil, eggs, vanilla extract, cream cheese, Swerve, and baking powder.

2. Combine all ingredients in a square baking dish and fold together.

3. Bake for 20 minutes at 320°F.

4. Allow to cool before slicing and serving.

• 228 calories • 23.1 grams of fat • 3.9 grams of carbohydrates • 4.8 grams of protein

20-minute prep time

Time to cook: 1 hour and 10 minutes

Number of servings: 10

• 12 cup butter • 2 oz chopped unsweetened chocolate • 12 cup almond flour • 14 cup cocoa powder

• 2 eggs • a pinch of salt

• 34 cup Swerve • 14 teaspoon vanilla extract • 14 cup chopped walnuts or pecans Filling for a cheesecake

• 1 pound softened cream cheese • 2 eggs • 12 cup Swerve • 14 cup heavy cream • 12 teaspoon vanilla extract

Instructions

1. Grease a springform pan and preheat the oven to 325F for the brownie base.

2. Melt the butter and chocolate in the microwave, then whisk until smooth.

3. In a mixing bowl, combine the cocoa powder, almond flour, and salt.

4. In a separate bowl, whisk together the eggs, vanilla, and Swerve until smooth.

5. Mix in the almond flour, then the chocolate-butter mixture, until smooth. Add the nuts and mix well. Cover the bottom of the prepared skillet with the flour mixture.

6. Bake for 12 to 18 minutes, or until set around the edges but still soft in the center. Cool.

7. Reduce the oven temperature to 300 degrees Fahrenheit for the filling.

8. In a mixing bowl, beat cream cheese with a mixer until smooth.

9. Mix in the cream, swerve, eggs, and vanilla until thoroughly combined.

10. Spread the filling over the crust of the cheesecake on a cookie sheet.

11. Bake for 35 to 45 minutes, or until just barely jiggling in the center.

12. Remove from oven and set aside to cool.

13. Chill for at least 3 hours in the refrigerator.

14. Serve.

Facts on Nutrition (Per Serving)

• Calories: 380

• Fat: 33g • Carbs: 6.8g • Protein: 8.7g

CHAPTER 4 DIABETIC BREAD RECIPES Lemon Bread from Starbucks

Prep time: 5 minutes 1 hour of cooking Servings: 15 Ingredients

• 6 eggs • 2 tbsp. unchilled cream cheese • 9 tbsp. butter • 1 tsp. vanilla • 2 tbsp. heavy whipping cream

• ½ tsp. of salt • 2/3 cup Monkfruit Classic • ½ cup + 2 tbsp. coconut flour • 1 ½ tsp. baking powder • 2 zest of 2 lemons (reserve 1 tsp. for the glaze) • 4 tsp. fresh lemon juice The Glaze • 2 tsp. freshly squeezed lemon juice • 2 tbsp. Monkfruit Powder • 1 tsp. lemon zest • 1 splash heavy whipping cream

Directions

1. Warm the oven to reach 325 degrees Fahrenheit. Prepare a bread pan using a layer of parchment baking paper.

2. Add the butter into a microwavable dish to melt. Let it cool.

3. Whisk the eggs, with the vanilla, heavy whipping cream, Monk fruit Classic, cream cheese, baking powder, and salt until combined.

4. Thoroughly mix in the coconut flour, melted butter, lemon zest, and juice to the mixture.

5. Scoop the batter into the prepared bread pan.

6. Bake it until the top of the bread is just beginning to brown and a toothpick inserted in the center comes out clean (55 min. to 1 hr.).

7. Prepare the glaze by combining the lemon juice with the Monkfruit Powder, lemon zest, and a splash of heavy whipping cream. Whisk until the glaze is creamy.

8. Empty the prepared glaze over the warm bread, spreading it out so that it covers the top

and runs down the sides to serve.

Nutrition Facts (Per Serving) • Calories: 121

• Fat: 10g • Carb: 3g • Protein: 8g

10 minute prep time 15-minute time to cook Servings: 10

• 6 ounces mozzarella cheese, shredded • 3 ounces almond meal

• 1 tbsp crushed garlic • 2 tbsp full fat cream cheese • 1 tsp baking powder

• 1 tbsp dried parsley • 1 medium egg • 1 pinch salt

1. Add every ingredient into a bowl, excluding the egg.

2. Lightly stir the mixture until combined.

3. Place bowl in a microwave and microwave for 1 minute on high.

4. Stir mixture and microwave for 30 seconds more.

5. Add the egg into the dough and gently stir until incorporated.

6. Add mixture onto a prepared baking tray and mold into a loaf shape.

7. Sprinkle any leftover cheese over the bread.

8. Bake loaf for 15 minutes at 425F, or until golden brown.

• Calories: 118

• Fat: 9.8g • Carbs: 2.4g • Protein: 6.2g

15 minute prep time Cook time: 35 minutes 16 portions

• 3 cups almond flour, blanched • 2 tbsp egg white protein powder

• ½ tsp baking soda

• 1 tsp cream of tartar • 6 large eggs • ¼ tsp sea salt • ½ tsp vanilla stevia • 1 tbsp lime zest • 1 cup frozen blueberries

1. Preheat oven to 350F and grease a loaf pan.

2. Add almond flour, protein powder, cream of tartar, baking soda, and salt in a food processor.

3. Pulse mixture to combine.

4. Continue to mix and add stevia, eggs, and lime zest into the food processor and pulse until you get a very smooth batter.

5. Add blueberries into the batter and stir until mixed.

6. Pour batter into the prepared loaf pan and transfer to the preheated oven.

7. Bake for 45 to 55 minutes, and cool for 2 hours.

8. Slice and serve.

• Calories: 231

• Fat: 18g • Carbs: 6.8g • Protein: 12g

10 minute prep time Cook time: 45 minutes 16 portions

• 2/3 cup coconut flour • ½ cup butter, melted • 3 tbsp coconut oil, melted • 1 1/3 cups almond flour • ½ tsp xanthan gum • 1 tsp baking powder

• 6 eggs • ½ tsp salt

1. Preheat the oven to 350F. Line a baking dish with parchment paper.

2. Beat the eggs until creamy.

3. Add in the flour (almond and coconut flour) and mix them for 1 minute.

4. Now add the xanthan gum, coconut oil, butter, baking powder, and salt and mix them until the dough turns thick.

5. Put the dough into the prepared bread loaf pan.

6. Bake for 40 to 45 minutes.

7. Cool, slice, and serve.

• Calories: 178

• Fat: 15g • Carbs: 5.1g • Protein: 5.8g

10 minute prep time Cook time: 45 minutes Servings: 10

• ½ cup coconut flour • 8 tbsp melted butter, cooled • 1 tsp baking powder

• 6 large eggs • 1 tsp garlic powder

• 2 tsp rosemary, dried • ¼ tsp salt • ½ tsp onion powder

1. Add coconut flour, baking powder, onion, garlic, rosemary, and salt into a bowl. Combine and mix well.

2. Add the eggs into another bowl and beat until bubbly on top.

3. Add melted butter into the bowl with the eggs and beat until mixed.

4. Gradually add the coconut flour mixture into the egg mixture. Mix with a hand mixer.

5. Preheat the oven to 350F.

6. Prepare a greased loaf pan.

7. Pour the soft dough into the prepared loaf pan and even the top with a spatula.

8. Transfer loaf pan into the preheated oven. Bake for 40 to 50 minutes.

9. Cool, slice, and serve.

• Calories: 157

• Fat: 12.5g • Carbs: 3.5g • Protein: 4.6g

10 minute prep time Cook time: 25 minutes Servings: 10

• ½ cup coconut flour • ½ tsp baking powder • ½ tsp baking soda • 1 tsp cinnamon • 1 tsp vinegar • 3 eggs • 1/8 tsp stevia • 2 tbsp Erythritol, powdered • 3 tbsp butter, salted • 1/3 cup Greek yogurt (you can use sour cream) • 2 tbsp water

1. Preheat the oven to 350F.

2. Use a parchment paper to line a greased loaf pan.

3. Combine the dry ingredients and whisk them until mixed.

4. Add unused ingredients and mix well. Taste for sweetness and adjust if necessary. Allow the dough to stand and mix again.

5. Pour the soft batter into the prepared loaf pan.

6. Bake for 25 to 30 minutes.

7. Remove, cool, and serve.

• Calories: 98

• Fat: 7.4g • Carbs: 2.5g • Protein: 3.9g

10 minute prep time 30 minute time to cook Servings: 4 • 1 tbsp butter, melted • 1 tbsp coconut oil, melted • 6 eggs • 1 tsp baking soda

• 2 tbsp ground flaxseed • 1 ½ tbsp psyllium husk powder • 5 tbsp coconut flour • 1 ½ cup almond flour

1. Preheat the oven to 400F.

2. Mix the eggs in a medium bowl for a few minutes.

3. Add in the butter and coconut oil. Mix once more for 1 minute.

4. Add the coconut flour, almond flour, baking soda, psyllium husk, and ground flaxseed to the mixture. Let sit for 15

minutes.

5. Lightly grease the loaf pan with coconut oil. Pour the mixture in the pan.

6. Place in the oven and bake until a toothpick inserted in it comes out dry, about 25 minutes.

• Calories: 458

• Fat: 38g • Carbs: 6.4g • Protein: 19g

10 minute prep time Cook time: 45 minutes Servings: 6

• ¼ cup butter, melted • 3 eggs • ¾ cup almond flour • ½ tsp baking powder

• ½ tsp Erythritol

1. Layer a loaf pan with parchment paper and preheat the oven to 350F.

2. Whisk the eggs and melted butter in a bowl.

3. Mix erythritol, almond flour, and baking powder in another bowl.

4. Combine the two mixtures to form a dough.

5. Transfer your dough to the loaf pan, place it in the oven.

6. Bake for about 45 minutes and remove it from the oven.

7. Cool, slice, and serve.

• There are 184 calories in a single serving of this recipe.

• Fat: 16.5g • Carbs: 4.6g • Protein: 5.9g

15 minute prep time 40-minute time to cook Servings: 16 slices • ½ tsp xanthan gum • ½ tsp salt • 2 tbsp coconut oil • ½ cup butter, melted • 1 tsp baking powder

• 2 cups of almond flour • 7 eggs

1. Preheat the oven to 355F.

2. Beat eggs in a bowl for at least 2 minutes until a thick foam appears.

3. Add coconut oil and butter to the eggs and continue to beat.

4. Cover a loaf pan with baking paper.

5. Pour the rest of the ingredients into the beaten eggs and butter and stir until thick.

6. Bake for about 40–45 minutes, until the control toothpick comes out dry.

• Calories: 236

• Fat: 23g • Carbs: 2.6g • Protein: 7g

Bagels filled with butter

10 minute prep time Cook time: 23 minutes Servings: 6

• ½ tsp baking soda

• 1 ¾ tbsp butter, unsalted and melted • 3 eggs, separated • ¼ tsp cream of tartar • 2 tbsp coconut flour, sifted • 1 ¾ tbsp cream cheese, full-fat and softened • 2 tsp Swerve sweetener, granulated • ¼ tsp salt • Coconut oil cooking spray

1. Preheat the oven to 300F. Coat a 6-cavity donut pan with coconut oil spray.

2. Divide the eggs between whites and yolks.

3. Blend the cream of tartar with the egg whites and pulse with a hand mixer for 5 minutes.

4. Combine the egg yolks with salt, baking soda, Swerve, coconut flour, melted butter, and cream cheese.

5. Gently blend the whipped eggs into the mix and blend well.

6. Fill the pan with the batter.

7. Bake in the oven for 23 minutes.

8. Cool and serve.

• Calories: 83

• Fat: 3g • Carbs: 1.6g • Protein: 6g

10 minute prep time 30 minute time to cook Servings: 6 • 1 cup boiling water or as needed • 2 cups almond flour • ½ cup ground flaxseed • 4 tbsp psyllium husk powder • 1 tbsp baking powder

• 2 tbsp olive oil • 2 eggs • 1 tbsp apple cider vinegar • ½ tsp salt

1. Preheat the oven to 350F.

2. In a medium bowl, mix well the almond flour, baking powder, psyllium husk powder, flax-seed flour, and salt.

3. Add the olive oil and eggs. Blend until the mixture resembles breadcrumbs, then mix in the apple cider vinegar.

4. Slowly add boiling water and mix into the mixture. Let stand for half an hour to firm up.

5. Line parchment paper over the baking tray.

6. Form the dough into a ball so that it fits in the palm of your hand.

7. Transfer dough balls on a baking tray and bake for 30 minutes, or until firm and golden.

• Calories: 301

• Fat: 24.1g • Carbs: 5.2g • Protein: 11g

Prep time: 5 minutes Cook time: 10 minutes Servings: 6 • ¼ cup almond flour • 1 ounce cream cheese • 1 cup shredded mozzarella

• ¼ cup ground flaxseed • ½ tsp baking soda

• 1 egg • Sesame seeds

1. Preheat the oven to 400F.

2. Cover a baking sheet with parchment paper. Remove the item from circulation.

3. In a bowl, add cream cheese and mozzarella and microwave for 1 minute or until melted.

4. Stir cheese mixture until a smooth consistency is achieved.

5. Add egg into the cheese mixture and stir to combine.

6. Add almond flour, ground flaxseed, and baking soda into another bowl and combine.

7. Add the egg and cheese mixture into the flour mixture and stir until a sticky dough is formed.

8. Mold the dough into six balls.

9. Sprinkle sesame seeds over each cheesy dough ball, place on the prepared baking sheet.

10. Transfer dough ball into the preheated oven and baking for 10 to 12 minutes, or until golden.

11. Cool and serve.

• Calories: 219

• Fat: 19g • Carbs: 2.3 • Protein: 10.7g

Prep time: 30 minutes 30 minute time to cook Servings: 6

• ¼ tsp ground turmeric • 1 medium cauliflower head • 2 eggs
• 2 tbsp coconut flour • Pinch of salt and pepper

1. Preheat the oven to 400F. Line a baking sheet with parchment paper.

2. Grind the cauliflower in a food processor until riced.

3. Add the riced cauliflower into a bowl with a tsp. of water, then cover with a plastic wrap with some holes on top.

4. Place the cauliflower bowl into the microwave and heat for 4 minutes.

5. Remove the plastic wrap and cool the cauliflower for 5 minutes. Then transfer into paper towels and squeeze out all excess moisture.

6. Pour the squeezed cauliflower into a bowl. Add eggs, flour, turmeric, salt, pepper, and mix.

7. Mold the mixture into 6 buns, then arrange on top of the baking sheet and fit into the oven.

8. Bake for 25 to 30 minutes.

9. Serve.

• There are 338 calories in 338 calories in 338 calories in 338 calories in 338

• 28g fat; 5g carbohydrate; 9g protein

15 minute prep time 15-minute time to cook Servings: 12

• 1 tbsp pretzel salt • 2 tbsp butter, melted • 2 tbsp warm water • 2 tsp dried yeast • 2 eggs • 2 tsp xanthan gum • 1 ½ cups almond flour • 4 tbsp cream cheese • 3 cups of shredded mozzarella cheese

1. Preheat the oven to 390F.

2. Melt the mozzarella cheese and cream cheese in the microwave.

3. Combine warm water with yeast and let sit for 2 minutes and activate.

4. Mix the almond meal and xanthan gum with a hand mixer.

5. Add yeast mixture, 1 tbsp. melted butter, and eggs and mix well.

6. Add in the melted cheese and knead the dough, about 5 to 10 minutes or until well combined.

7. Divide into 12 balls while the dough is still warm, then roll into a long, thin log and then twist to form a pretzel shape.

8. Transfer onto a lined cookie sheet, leaving small space between them.

9. Brush the remaining butter on top the pretzels and sprinkle with the salt.

10. Bake for 12 to 15 minutes in the oven or until golden brown.

• Calories: 217

• Fat: 17g • Carbs: 3g • Protein: 11g

15 minute prep time 30 minute time to cook Servings: 6 • 2 tbsp coconut flour • 3 tbsp flaxseed meal

• ½ tsp baking powder

• 4 eggs, separated • 1 tsp dried minced onion

1. Preheat the oven to 325F. Grease a donut pan with cooking spray.

2. Sift the flax meal, coconut flour, minced onion, and baking powder.

3. Whip the egg whites until foamy. Slowly whisk in the yolks and dry mixture. Let the dough thicken for 5 to 10 minutes.

4. Scoop into the molds and sprinkle with a portion of dried onion to your liking.

5. Bake for 30 minutes, or until golden brown.

6. Cool and serve.

• Calories: 78

• Fat: 5g • Carbs: 1.5g • Protein: 5g

Cowboy Cookies are the best.

20-minute prep time 15-minute time to cook 8 people

• 2 large eggs • 2 cups almond flour • 2 tsp baking powder • 1 tsp baking soda • 1 cup butter, softened • 1 cup swerve white sugar • 1 cup swerve brown sugar • 1 tbsp vanilla extract • 1 tbsp cinnamon powder

• 1 cup sugar-free chocolate chips

• 1 cup peanut butter chips

• 2 cups golden flaxseed meal

• 1 ½ cups coconut flakes • 2 cups chopped walnuts • 1 tsp salt

1. Preheat oven to 380 F. Line a baking sheet with parchment paper.

2. In a large bowl, using a hand mixer, cream the butter and swerve white and brown sugar until light and fluffy. Slowly, beat in the vanilla and eggs until smooth.

3. In a separate bowl, mix almond flour, baking powder, baking soda, cinnamon, and salt.

4. Combine both mixtures and fold in the chocolate chips, peanut butter chips, flaxseed meal, coconut flaxes, and walnuts.

5. Roll the dough into 1 ½-inch balls and arrange on the baking sheet at 2inch intervals.

6. Bake for 10 to 12 minutes. Or until lightly golden.

7. Serve.

• Calories: 290

• Fat: 32.8g • Carb: 4.6g • Protein: 16g

10 minute prep time 15-minute time to cook Servings: 30

• 1 ½ cup almond flour • ¼ tsp garlic powder • ½ tsp onion powder • ½ tsp thyme • ¼ tsp basil • ¼ tsp oregano • ¾ tsp salt • 1 egg • 2 tbsp olive oil

1. Preheat the oven to 350F. Line a baking sheet with parchment paper. Remove the item from circulation.

2. Combine all the cracker ingredients in a food processor until dough forms.

3. Mold the dough into a smooth log and slice into thin crackers. Arrange the crackers onto the prepared baking sheet and bake for 10 to 15 minutes.

4. Cool and serve.

• Calories: 63.5 • Fat: 5.8g • Carbs: 1.8g • Protein: 2.2g

10 minute prep time 15-minute time to cook Servings: 4 • 1 egg • 1 cup ground pecans • 2 tbsp sweetener • ¼ tsp baking soda • 1 tbsp butter • 4 walnuts, halved

1. Mix all ingredients, except the walnuts, until well combined.

2. Make balls out of the mixture and press them with your thumb onto a lined cookie sheet. Top each cookie with a walnut half.

3. Bake for about 12 minutes in a preheated to 340 F oven.

• Calories: 163

• Fat: 13g • Carb: 2.4g • Protein: 3.2g

10 minute prep time 20-minute cook time Servings: 40 crackers

• 1 cup almond flour • ¼ tsp baking soda • ¼ tsp salt • 1/8 tsp black pepper • 3 tbsp sesame seeds • 1 egg, beaten • Salt and pepper to taste

1. Preheat your oven to 350 °F.

2. Line two baking sheets with parchment paper and keep them on the side.

3. Mix the dry ingredients into a large bowl and add egg, mix well and form a dough.

4. Divide dough into two balls.

5. Roll out the dough. It is more convenient to do this by placing the dough between two sheets of parchment paper.

6. Cut into crackers and transfer them to prep a baking sheet.

7. Bake for 15-20 minutes.

8. Repeat until all the dough has been used up Leave crackers to cool and serve.

9. Enjoy!

• Calories: 170

• Fat: 18g • Carb: 3.4g • Protein: 10.1g

10 minute prep time Cook time: 10 minutes Servings: 18

• ½ cup butter, plus more for greasing the baking sheet • ½ cup granulated sweetener • 1 tsp vanilla extract • 1 ½ cups almond flour • ½ cup ground hazelnuts • A pinch of sea salt

1. In a bowl, cream together the vanilla, sweetener, and butter until well blended.

2. Stir in salt, ground hazelnuts, and flour and make a dough.

3. Roll the dough into a 2-inch cylinder. Wrap it in plastic wrap. For complete cooling place the dough in the refrigerator for at least 30 minutes.

4. Preheat the oven to 350F. Line a baking sheet with parchment paper. Lightly grease the paper with butter. Remove the item from circulation.

5. Unwrap the chilled cylinder. Slice the dough into 18 cookies. Place the cookies on the baking sheet.

6. Bake for 10 minutes. Or until firm and lightly browned.

7. Cool and serve.

• Calories: 105

• Fat: 10g • Carbs: 2g • Protein: 3g

10 minute prep time 20-minute cook time Servings: 15 • 2/3 cup nut butter of choice • 5 tbsp coconut flour • 2/3 cup Erythritol • 1 egg • 1/3 cup butter, melted • 1/3 cup dark chocolate chips or chunks (sugar-free)

1. Preheat the oven to 350F.

2. Grease a baking sheet.

3. In a bowl, combine the nut butter, flour, egg, Erythritol and butter. Mix well.

4. Add the sugar-free chocolate chips and make the dough.

5. Freeze the dough for 10 minutes (the freezer will help you).

6. Spoon the chilled dough in the freezer onto the cookie sheet.

7. Bake until browned. About 15 to 20 minutes.

8. Remove from oven. Cool completely.

• Calories: 120

• Fat: 11g • Carbs: 5g • Protein: 4g

10 minute prep time Cook time: 10 minutes Servings: 24

• 4 ounces butter, melted • 2 ounces full fat cream cheese • 1 egg • 1-ounce coconut flour • ½ tsp. baking powder • ½ tsp. baking soda • ¼ tsp. liquid stevia extract • ½ tsp. xanthan gum • ½ tsp. vanilla extract

1. Preheat the oven to 350F. Line a cookie sheet with parchment paper.

2. In a clean bowl mix together the butter and cream cheese.

3. In another bowl, mix the coconut flour, baking powder, xanthan gum, and baking soda.

4. In another bowl, add sugar substitute and vanilla to the egg and beat well.

5. Add the dry ingredients to the butter and cream cheese and mix well.

6. Stir in the egg mixture and combine everything well together.

7. Drop small spoonful's of the mixture onto the prepared sheet and bake for 8 to 10 minutes.

8. Cool and serve .

• Calories: 51

• Fat: 5g • Carbs: 0.8g • Protein: 0.9g

10 minute prep time 15-minute time to cook Servings: 20 • 2 ½ cups almond flour • ½ cup peanut butter • ¼ cup coconut oil • ¼ cup Erythritol • 3 tbsp. maple syrup • 1 tbsp. vanilla extract • 1 ½ tsp. baking powder • ½ tsp. salt • 2 to 3 dark chocolate bars

1. Whisk the wet ingredients together.

2. Separately, mix the dry ingredients. Sift them into the wet ingredients. Mix well. Refrigerate for 20 to 30 minutes.

3. Break the dark chocolate bars into small squares.

4. From small balls of dough and press flat.

5. Add 1 to 2 pieces of chocolate in the middle and seal together into a ball.

6. Place on a parchment-paper-lined cookie tray and bake at 350F for 15 minutes.

• Calories: 150

• Fat: 14g • Carbs: 2.7g • Protein: 4.5g

Truffles de cacao

10 minute prep time Cook time: 6 minutes Servings: 22

• 1 cup sugar-free chocolate chips

• 2 tbsp butter • 2/3 cup heavy cream • 2 tsp brandy • 2 tbsp swerve • ¼ tsp vanilla extract • Cocoa powder to roll the truffles

1. Add the heavy cream to a bowl.

2. Add swerve, butter, chocolate chips, and stir. Put in the microwave. Heat for 1 minute.

3. Set aside for 5 minutes. Stir well. Mix with brandy and vanilla extract.

4. Stir again the chocolate mix. Set aside in the refrigerator for 2 hours.

5. Transform the future truffle into balls.

6. Roll them in cocoa powder and serve.

• Calories: 68

• Fat: 4.4g • Carbs: 6.1g • Protein: 1.2g

Chapter Nine

Healthy Dessert

10 minute prep time 20-minute cook time 4 people

• 2 tbsp unsweetened cocoa powder • ½ tsp vanilla extract • ½ cup Erythritol • 1 tbsp xanthan gum mixed in • 1 tbsp water • A pinch salt • 6 tbsp cool water • 2 ½ tsp gelatin powder Dusting

• 1 tbsp unsweetened cocoa powder • 1 tbsp swerve confectioner's sugar

1. Grease a lined with parchment paper loaf pan with cooking spray; set aside.

2. Mix the erythritol, 2 tbsp of water, xanthan gum mixture and salt in a saucepan. Place the pan over high heat and

bring to a boil. Insert a thermometer and let the ingredients simmer at 220 F, for 8 minutes.

3. Add 2 tbsp of water and sprinkle the gelatin on top, in a small bowl. Let sit to dissolve for 5 minutes. While the gelatin dissolves, pour the remaining water in a small bowl and heat in the microwave for 30 seconds. Stir in cocoa powder and mix it into the gelatin.

4. When the erythritol solution has hit the right temperature, gradually pour it directly into the gelatin mixture, stirring continuously. Beat for 12 minutes to get a light and fluffy consistency.

5. Then, stir in the vanilla and pour the blend into the loaf pan. Let the marshmallows set for 3 hours in the fridge.

6. Use an oiled knife to cut into cubes and place them on a plate.

7. Mix the remaining cocoa powder and confectioner's sugar together. Sift it over the marshmallows.

• Calories: 94

• Fat: 3.8g

• Carb: 3.6g • Protein: 2.2g

Prep time: 5 minutes + Cooling Cook time: 10 minutes Servings: 4 • 2 cups raw cashew nuts • 2 tbsp flax seed • 1 ½ cups blueberry preserves, sugar-free • 3 tbsp Xylitol • 10 oz unsweetened chocolate chips

• 3 tbsp olive oil

1. Grind the cashew nuts and flax seeds in a blender for 50 seconds until smoothly crushed; add the blueberries and 2 tbsp of xylitol. Process further for 1 minute until well combined.

2. Form 1-inch balls of the mixture.

3. Line a baking sheet with parchment paper. Place the balls on the baking sheet. Freeze for 1 hour or until firmed up.

4. In a microwave, melt the chocolate chips, oil and the remaining xylitol, for 95 seconds.

5. Toss the truffles to coat in the chocolate mixture, put on the baking sheet, and freeze up for at least 3 hours.

• Calories: 264

• Fat: 19.2g • Carb: 4.2g • Protein: 10.2g

10 minute prep time Cook time: 10 minutes Servings: 20 • 2 tbsp Stevia • 4 egg whites • 2 cups coconut, shredded • 1 tsp vanilla extract

1. Mix egg whites with stevia in a bowl and beat with a mixer.

2. Add vanilla extract and coconut and stir.

3. Roll mixture into small balls. Place them on a lined baking sheet.

4. Place in the oven at 350°F. Bake for 10 minutes.

5. Cool and serve.

• Calories: 39

• Fat: 2.7g • Carbs: 1.3g • Protein: 1.2g

10 minute prep time Cook time: 10 minutes Servings: 12

• 3 fresh strawberries • ½ tsp vanilla • ¾ cup Swerve • ½ cup butter • 8 oz. cream cheese, softened

1. Put all candy ingredients into the food processor. Blend until the mixture is completely smooth.

2. Pour mixture into the silicone candy mold and place it in the refrigerator for 2 hours or until candy is hardened.

3. Serve.

• Calories: 136

• Fat: 14.2g • Carbs: 0.9g • Protein: 1.5g

Prep time: 1 hour 15 minutes Cook time: 0 minute Servings: 9 Ingredients

• 1 cup coconut oil • 1 cup cocoa powder • ¼ cup powdered Erythritol • 1 tsp vanilla bean powder

• 15 drops Stevia extract • Salt to taste • ¼ cup coconut butter, chilled

Instructions

1. Melt coconut oil in a microwave. Combine with the next four ingredients.

2. Spoon about ½ of the chocolate mixture into silicone molds. Refrigerate for 15 minutes.

3. Remove from the refrigerator and add ½ teaspoon coconut butter into each mold.

4. Top with the remaining chocolate mixture and refrigerate for 40 minutes.

5. Serve.

Facts on Nutrition (Per Serving)

• Calories: 76

• Fat: 7.7g • Carbs: 1g • Protein: 1g

Fat Bombs (Red Velvet)

Prep time: 55 minutes Cook time: 0 minute Servings: 24
Ingredients

• 3.5 oz. 90 percent dark chocolate • 4.5 oz. cream cheese, softened • 3.5 oz. butter, softened • 1 tsp Stevia • 1 tsp vanilla extract • 4 drops red food coloring • ⅓ cup heavy cream, whipped

Instructions

1. Melt chocolate in the microwave.

2. Combine the remaining ingredients, except for the whipped cream, with a hand mixer.

3. Add the melted chocolate and mix well.

4. Fill a piping bag with the bombs mixture and transfer the fat bomb mixture onto a lined tray.

5. Refrigerate for 40 minutes.

6. Top with whipped cream.

7. Cut into servings and serve.

Nutrition Facts (Per Serving) • Calories: 85

• Fat: 9g • Carbs: 2g • Protein: 1.1g

50-minute prep time Minutes to prepare: 0
Ingredients/Servings: 14

• 1 cup unsalted macadamia nuts • 14 cup extra-virgin coconut oil • 14 cup butter • 2 tbsp powdered Erythritol

Instructions

In a blender, pulverize the macadamia nuts. Softened butter and coconut oil are combined with them.

2. Combine the rest of the ingredients in a large mixing bowl. Make a thorough mixture.

3. Pour 112 tablespoons of the mixture into each of 12 mini-muffin cups.

4. Allow 30 minutes in the refrigerator before serving.

Nutritional Information (Per Serving)

• There are 132 calories in a single serving of this dish.

• 14.4g fat; 4g carbohydrate; 2g protein

1 hour and 15 minutes to prepare 0 minutes of cooking 16 portions

• 7 oz. softened coconut butter • 14 cup extra-virgin coconut oil

In a large mixing bowl, combine all of the ingredients.

2. Fill each small muffin paper cup with 1 tablespoon of the coconut mixture and set on a tray.

3. Allow 1 hour to chill before serving.

• There are 112 calories in this dish.

• 11.9 g fat • 3 g carbohydrates • 1 g protein

2 hours and 50 minutes of prep time Minutes to prepare: 0 Ingredients/Servings: 24

• 12 cup butter • 12 cup coconut oil • 12 cup sour cream

2 tbsp erythritol • 25 drops liquid stevia • 2 tbsp cocoa powder • 1 tsp vanilla extract

Instructions

1. In a large mixing bowl, whisk together the first six ingredients.

2. Separate the ingredients into three bowls. In the first bowl, combine cocoa powder, strawberries, and vanilla extract. In the second bowl, combine cocoa powder, strawberries, and vanilla extract.

3. Fill fat bomb molds with cocoa powder mixture.

4. Chill for 30 minutes in the freezer. To make a second layer, repeat with the vanilla mixture.

5. Allow 30 minutes to freeze the vanilla mixture.

6. Lastly, add the strawberry mixture to the mix.

7. Return everything to the freezer for at least one hour.

8. Serve.

Facts on Nutrition (Per Serving)

• 102 Calories

• 11 g fat • 1.1 g carbohydrate • 1.1 g protein

15 minute prep time Minutes to prepare: 0
Ingredients/Servings: 6

• 3 tablespoons coconut oil • 5 tablespoons butter

2 tbsp blueberry syrup (sugar-free) + 2 tbsp cocoa powder

Instructions

1. In a saucepan over low heat, combine all bomb ingredients until well combined.

2. Freeze for at least 3 hours in silicone molds.

3. Serve.

Facts on Nutrition (Per Serving)

• There are 148 calories in a single serving of this dish.

• 17 grams of fat • 1 gram of carbohydrates • 0.6 grams of protein

1 hour and 5 minutes to prepare 5 minutes to prepare
Number of servings: 15

• 1.7 oz unsalted butter • 14 oz ricotta cheese • 20 drops liquid stevia • 1 tbsp psyllium husks • 13 cup shredded coconut • 34 tsp cardamom • 12 tsp vanilla extract • 2 tbsp coconut oil

Instructions

1. Melt the butter in a saucepan and add the ricotta cheese.

2. Toss all of the ingredients together, except the shredded coconut and almonds, in a large mixing bowl. Combine the ingredients in a mixing bowl and stir in the melted cheese. Cool.

3. Form the mixture into balls and stuff each one with an almond.

4. Cover the balls with a thick layer of grated coconut.

5. Allow 30 minutes in the refrigerator before serving.

6. Serve.

Facts on Nutrition (Per Serving)

• 136 calories per serving • 13 grams of fat • 2 grams of carbohydrates • 3 grams of protein

3 hr. 15 min. prep time Minutes to prepare: 0
Ingredients/Servings: 12

• 14 cup coconut oil • 14 cup almond butter • 2 tsp rum extract • 12 drops liquid Stevia

Instructions

1. In a saucepan over medium heat, combine all ingredients, except the cocoa powder. Stir the ingredients frequently until they have melted. Remove the heat from the room.

2. Stir in the cocoa powder thoroughly.

3. Pour the mixture into 12 silicone candy molds or ice cube trays with silicone bottoms.

4. Allow to set in the freezer for at least an hour.

5. Serve.

Facts on Nutrition (Per Serving)

• There are 75 calories in this recipe.

• 7 grams of fat • 2 grams of carbohydrates • 2 grams of protein

Muffins filled with pumpkin

10 minute prep time 18-minute time to cook 5 people

• 12 tsp salt • 12 tsp baking powder • 1 egg • 1 tbsp vanilla extract • 1 tbsp apple cider vinegar

1. Preheat oven to 350 degrees Fahrenheit (180 degrees Celsius).

2. Combine all ingredients in this recipe, except the almonds, in a mixing bowl.

3. Preheat the oven to 350°F and prepare a 5-portion muffin pan. Spritz with a little bit of extra virgin olive oil.

4. Add crushed almonds as a finishing touch.

5. Preheat oven to 350°F and bake for 15–18 minutes.

• There are 185 calories in a single serving of this dish.

• 13.5 grams of fat • 3.5 grams of carbohydrates • 7.4 grams of protein

5 minutes to prepare 25-minute time to cook 8 servings • 4 large eggs • 1 tsp Stevia • 12 tbsp vanilla extract • 12 cup coconut flour • 14 cup melted coconut oil • 1 tbsp baking powder • 1 pinch salt • 14 tbsp cloves powder • 1/3 cup coconut milk

Preheat oven to 325 degrees Fahrenheit.

2. In a mixing bowl, whisk together the eggs, vanilla extract, and stevia.

3. Once the eggs have been thoroughly beaten, stir in the coconut flour, oil, baking powder, salt, and clove powder, as well as the coconut milk.

4. Pour the batter into the greased muffin tin once all of the ingredients have been thoroughly combined.

5. Bake for about 25 minutes, or until muffins are golden brown.

6. Place cranberries and rosemary on top of each muffin and top with chilled heavy whipped cream.

7. Enjoy as a Christmas snack with a cup of keto creamy coffee.

• There are 174 calories in a single serving of this recipe.

16.3 grams of fat, 3.6 grams of carbohydrates, and 3.8 grams of protein

5 minutes to prepare 25-minute time to cook 12 servings • 8 eggs • 8 ounces cream cheese • 2 tablespoons whey protein • 4 tablespoons melted butter

1. Preheat oven to 350 degrees Fahrenheit (180 degrees Celsius).

2. In a mixing bowl, combine the melted butter and the cream cheese.

3. Using a hand mixer, thoroughly combine the whey protein and eggs in the mixing bowl.

4. Pour the batter into a muffin pan that has been prepared and placed in the oven.

5. Preheat the oven to 350°F and bake for 25 minutes.

6. Serve.

• There are 165 calories in a single serving of this dish.

• 13.6 g fat • 1.5 g carbohydrate • 9.6 g protein

10 minute prep time 20-minute cook time • 6 ounces melted coconut oil • 6 eggs • 3 ounces cocoa powder • 12 servings

• 2 tbsp Swerve • 2 tbsp vanilla extract • 12 tbsp baking powder • 4 oz cream cheese

1. In a mixing bowl, whisk together the eggs, coconut oil, cocoa powder, baking powder, vanilla extract, cream cheese, and Swerve.

2. Transfer to a baking dish that has been lined with parchment paper.

3. Preheat the oven to 350 degrees Fahrenheit (180 degrees Celsius). 20 minutes in the oven

4. Allow to cool completely before cutting into rectangles.

5. Serve.

• There are 202 calories in a single serving of this dish.

• 20.6 grams of fat • 4.3 grams of carbohydrates • 4.1 grams of protein

10 minute prep time 45-minute time to cook 8 people

• cocoa powder (14 cup)

• 6 tbsp coconut flour • 2 tsp baking powder • 12 cup water • 12 cup peanut butter

1. Preheat oven to 350 degrees Fahrenheit (180 degrees Celsius).

2. Combine the peanut butter, stevia, and warm water in a mixing bowl.

3. Mix the cocoa powder, baking powder, and flour together in a separate bowl.

4. Combine the two batters and pour into a greased baking pan.

5. Preheat oven to 350°F and bake 45 minutes.

6. Serve.

• There are 143 calories in this recipe.

• 9 g fat • 6 g carbohydrate • 10 g protein

Cupcakes containing blueberries

10 minute prep time 20-minute cook time 12 portions

• 6 large eggs • 1 tsp baking powder • 2 tbsp lemon zest • 1 tsp vanilla extract • 2 tbsp lemon juice • 5 12 oz softened butter • 1 344 oz coconut flour • 4 12 oz blueberries • Cupcake liners

1. In a bowl, combine everything except the eggs and blueberries.

2. Crack the eggs into the mixture and thoroughly combine them. Carry on with the remaining eggs in a similar manner.

3. Fill each cupcake liner halfway with blueberries.

4. Fill each cupcake tin halfway with batter. 34% of the way up

5. Bake for 10 to 15 minutes at 350 degrees Fahrenheit.

6. Allow to cool before eating.

• There are 138 calories in a single serving of this dish.

11.4 g fat, 2.6 g carbs, and 4.4 g protein

15 minute prep time 30 minute time to cook 6 people

• 3 tbsp coconut flour • 1 tsp pumpkin pie spice

• baking soda (14 tsp)

• Pinch of salt\s• ¾ cup pumpkin puree\s• 1/3 cup Swerve\s• ¼ cup heavy whipping cream\s• 1 egg\s• ½ tsp vanilla

1. Line 6 muffin cups with parchment paper and preheat the oven to 350F.

2. In a bowl, whisk together the salt, baking soda, baking powder, pumpkin pie spice, and coconut flour.

3. In another bowl, whisk egg, vanilla, cream, sweetener, and pumpkin puree until mixed. Whisk in dry ingredients.

4. Pour into the muffin cups. Bake until just puffed and almost set, about 25 to 30 minutes.

5. Remove and cool.

6. Refrigerate for about 1 hour.

7. Top with whipped cream and serve.

• Calories: 70

• Fat: 4.1g\s• Carbs: 5.1g\s• Protein: 1.7g

10 minute prep time 15-minute time to cook 6 people

• ½ tsp salt\s• 1 cup flaxseed meal

• ¼ cup cocoa powder\s• 1 tbsp cinnamon\s• ½ tbsp baking powder\s• 2 tbsp coconut oil\s• 1 egg\s• ¼ cup sugar-free caramel syrup\s• 1 tsp vanilla extract\s• ½ cup pumpkin puree\s• ½ cup slivered almonds\s• 1 tsp apple cider vinegar

1. Preheat oven to 350 degrees Fahrenheit (180 degrees Celsius).

2. Put all everything (except the almonds) in a bowl and mix well.

3. Place 6 paper liners in the muffin tin and add ¼-cup batter to each one.

4. Sprinkle almonds and press gently.

5. Bake for 15 minutes. Or until the top is set.

• Calories: 183

• Fat: 13g\s• Carbs: 4.4g\s• Protein: 7g

Prep time: 3 minutes Cook time: 12 minutes Servings: 1\s• 1 egg\s• 2 tsp coconut flour\s• ¼ tsp baking powder\s• ¼ tsp sweetener\s• 2 tbsp shredded coconut\s• Coconut oil spray for muffin cups\s• Salt to taste

1. Whisk all ingredients to combine.

2. Grease muffin cups and pour in the dough.

3. Bake at 400°F for 12 minutes.

• Calories: 113

• Fat: 6g\s• Carbs: 5g\s• Protein: 7g

Cherries and Chocolate Mousse

10 minute prep time 30 minute time to cook 4 people

• 12 oz unsweetened dark chocolate\s• 8 eggs, separated into yolks and whites\s• 2 tbsp salt\s• ¾ cup swerve sugar\s• ½ cup olive oil\s• 3 tbsp brewed coffee Cherries

• 1 cup cherries, pitted and halved\s• ½ stick cinnamon\s• ½ cup swerve sugar\s• ½ cup water\s• ½ lime, juiced

1. In a bowl, add the chocolate and melt in the microwave for 95 seconds.

2. In a separate bowl, whisk the yolks with half of the swerve sugar until a pale yellow has formed, then, beat in the salt, olive oil, and coffee. Mix in the melted chocolate until smooth.

3. In a third bowl, whisk the whites with the hand mixer until a soft peak has formed. Sprinkle the remaining swerve sugar over and gently fold in with a spatula. Fetch a tablespoon of the chocolate mixture and fold in to combine. Pour in the remaining chocolate mixture and whisk to mix.

4. Ladle the mousse into ramekins, cover with plastic wrap, and refrigerate overnight.

5. The next day, pour ½ cup of water, ½ cup of swerve, ½ stick cinnamon, and lime juice in a saucepan and bring to a simmer for 4 minutes, stirring to ensure the swerve has dissolved and a syrup has formed.

6. Add cherries and poach in the sweetened water for 20 minutes until soft.

7. Turn heat off and discard the cinnamon stick.

8. Spoon a plum each with syrup on the chocolate mousse and serve.

• Calories: 248

• Fat: 23g\s• Carb: 4.1g\s• Protein: 12g

10 minute prep time Cook time: 10 minutes 4 people

• 1 2/3 cup coconut milk\s• 1 tbsp gelatin\s• 6 tbsp Swerve\s• 3 egg yolks\s• ½ tsp vanilla extract

1. In a bowl, mix gelatin with 1 Tbsp. coconut milk, stir well, and set aside.

2. Put the rest of the milk into a pan and heat over medium heat.

3. Add Swerve, stir, and cook for 5 minutes.

4. In a bowl, mix egg yolks with the hot coconut milk and vanilla extract. Stir well and return everything to the pan.

5. Cook for 4 minutes add gelatin and stir well.

6. Divide this into 4 ramekins and keep in the fridge until ready to serve.

• Calories: 134

• Fat: 2.2g\s• Carbs: 2.1g\s• Protein: 2g

10 minute prep time 20-minute cook time Servings: 3\sFor the mousse\s• 1 cup cold heavy cream

• 8 oz cream cheese\s• ¼ cup swerve sugar\s• 1 tsp vanilla extract\s• ½ lemon, juiced For the caramel nuts\s• 1 cup walnuts, chopped\s• 2/3 cup swerve brown sugar\s• A pinch salt

1. In a stand mixer, beat cream cheese and heavy cream until creamy. Add vanilla, swerve sugar, and lemon juice until smooth.

2. Divide the mixture between 4 dessert cups. Cover with plastic wrap, and refrigerate for at least 2 hours.

3. For the caramel walnuts: Add swerve sugar to a large skillet and cook over medium heat with frequent stirring until melted and golden brown. Mix in 2 tbsp of water and salt and cook further until syrupy and slightly thickened.

4. Turn the heat off and quickly mix in the walnuts until well coated in the caramel; let sit for 5 minutes.

5. Remove the mousse from the fridge and top with the caramel walnuts.

6. Serve immediately.

• There are 315 calories in a single serving of this dish.

• Fat: 26.8g • Carb: 4.2g • Protein: 7.2g

5 minutes to prepare Cook time: 0 minutes 4 people

• 4 ounces cream cheese, softened • ½ cup unsalted butter, softened • 2 tbsp granulated Erythritol • ½ large avocado, peeled and chopped • 2 tbsp unsweetened cocoa powder • 2/3 cup heavy cream

1. In a bowl, mix butter, cream cheese, and Erythritol. Beat until light and fluffy.

2. Add cocoa powder and avocado, beat until smooth. Stir in heavy cream.

3. Divide into 4 serving bowls and refrigerate until chilled. About 30 minutes.

4. Serve.

• Calories: 387

• Fat: 42g • Carbs: 3.1g • Protein: 3.8g

Cereal and Walnut Chaffle

10 minute prep time Cook time: 10 minutes Servings: 2

• 15-20 drops cereal flavoring • ¼ tsp. baking powder • 1 tsp. granulated swerve • 1/8 tsp. Xanthan gum • 1 tbsp. butter (melted) • ½ tsp. coconut flour • 2 tbsp. toasted walnut (chopped) • 1 tbsp. cream cheese • 2 tbsp. almond flour • 1 large egg (beaten) • ¼ tsp. cinnamon • 1/8 tsp. nutmeg

1. Plug the waffle maker to preheat it and spray it with a non-stick spray.

2. In a mixing bowl, whisk together the egg, cereal flavoring, cream cheese and butter.

3. In another mixing bowl, combine the coconut flour, almond flour, cinnamon, nutmeg, swerve, xanthan gum and baking powder.

4. Pour the egg mixture into the flour mixture and mix until you form a smooth batter.

5. Fold in the chopped walnuts.

6. Pour in an appropriate amount of batter into the waffle maker and spread out the batter to the edges to cover all the holes on the waffle maker.

7. Close the waffle maker and cook for about 3 minutes or according to your waffle maker's settings.

8. After the cooking cycle, use a plastic or silicone utensil to remove the chaffle from the waffle maker.

9. Repeat steps 6 to 8 until you have cooked all the batter into chaffles.

10. Serve and top with sour cream or heavy cream.

• Calories: 274

• Fat: 19g

• Carb: 4.6g • Protein: 18g

5 minutes to prepare Cook time: 10 minutes Servings: 2 • 1 egg, lightly beaten • ½ cup mozzarella cheese, shredded • ½ tsp psyllium husk powder

• ¼ tsp garlic powder

1. Preheat your waffle maker.

2. Whisk egg in a bowl with remaining ingredients until well combined.

3. Spray waffle maker with cooking spray.

4. Pour 1/2 of batter in the hot waffle maker and cook until golden brown. Repeat with the remaining batter.

5. Servings and enjoy.

• Calories: 134

• Fat: 5.8g • Carbs: 2.6g • Protein: 4.7g

10 minute prep time 20-minute cook time
Ingredients/Servings: 4

Cannoli topping • 2 tbsp. granulated swerve • 4 tbsp. cream cheese • ¼ tsp. vanilla extract • ¼ tsp. cinnamon • 6 tbsp. Ricotta cheese • 1 tsp. lemon juice Chaffle • 3 tbsp. almond flour • 1 tbsp. Swerve

• 1 egg • 1/8 tsp. baking powder • ¾ tbsp. butter (melted) • ½ tsp. nutmeg • 1 tbsp. sugar-free chocolate chips

• 1/8 tsp. vanilla extract

Directions

1. Plug the waffle maker to preheat it and spray it with a non-stick spray.

2. In a mixing bowl, whisk together the egg, butter and vanilla extract.

3. In another mixing bowl, combine the almond flour, baking powder, nutmeg, chocolate chips and swerve.

4. Pour the egg mixture into the flour mixture and mix until the ingredients are well combined and you have formed a smooth batter.

5. Fill your waffle maker with an appropriate amount of batter and spread out the batter to the edges to cover all the holes on the waffle maker.

6. Close the waffle maker and cook for about 4 minutes or according to the waffle maker's settings.

7. After the baking cycle, remove the chaffle from the waffle maker with a plastic or silicone utensil.

8. Repeat steps 5 to 7 until you have cooked all the batter into waffles.

9. For the topping, pour the cream cheese into a blender and add the ricotta, lemon juice, cinnamon, vanilla and swerve sweetener. Blend until smooth and fluffy.

10. Spread the cream over the chaffles and enjoy.

Facts on Nutrition (Per Serving)

• Calories: 104

• Fat: 9g • Carb: 4g • Protein: 13g

SWEET RECIPES Coconut Panna Cotta Caramel

10 minute prep time 5 minutes to prepare
Ingredients/Servings: 4

• 4 eggs • 1/3 cup Erythritol, for caramel • 2 cups coconut milk
• 1 tbsp vanilla extract • 1 tbsp lemon zest • ½ cup Erythritol,
for custard • 2 cup heavy whipping cream

• Mint leaves, to serve Instructions

1. In a deep pan, heat the erythritol for the caramel. Add two tablespoons of water and bring to a boil. Lower the heat and cook until the caramel turns to a golden brown color.

2. Divide between 4 metal tins, set aside and let cool.

3. In a bowl, mix the eggs, remaining erythritol, lemon zest, and vanilla.

4. Beat in the coconut milk until well combined.

5. Pour the custard into each caramel-lined ramekin and place them into a deep baking tin. Fill over the way with the remaining hot water.

6. Bake at 350 F for around 45 minutes. Carefully, take out the ramekins with tongs and refrigerate for at least 3 hours. Run a knife slowly around the edges to invert onto a dish.

7. Serve with dollops of whipped cream and scattered with mint leaves.

Facts on Nutrition (Per Serving)

• Calories: 268 • Fat: 20.8g • Carb: 2.6g • Protein: 6.5g

Time to prepare: 10 minutes plus time to cool Cook time: 10 minutes

Servings: 2

• 1 cup yogurt, full-fat • 2 tsp Xylitol • 2 tbsp chia seeds • 1 cup fresh strawberries, sliced • 1 tbsp lemon zest • Mint leaves, to serve

1. In a bowl, combine the yogurt and xylitol together. Add in the chia seeds and stir.

2. Reserve a couple of strawberries for garnish, and mash the remaining ones with a fork until pureed.

3. Stir in the yogurt mixture and refrigerate for 45 minutes.

4. Once cooled, divide the mixture between glasses.

5. Top each with the reserved slices of strawberries, mint leaves, and lemon zest.

• Calories: 190

• Fat: 10.8g • Carb: 3.2g • Protein: 6.2g

5 minutes to prepare Cook time: 10 minutes Servings: 3 • 1 cup ricotta cheese • 2 cups strawberries, chopped • 2 tbsp sugar-free maple syrup • 2 tbsp balsamic vinegar

1. Distribute half of the strawberries between 4 small glasses and top with ricotta cheese.

2. Drizzle with maple syrup, balsamic vinegar and finish with the remaining strawberries.

3. Serve.

• Calories: 159

• Fat: 8g • Carb: 3.1g • Protein: 6.2g

5 minutes to prepare Minutes to prepare: 0 4 people

• ¼ cup fresh cranberries • 2 tbsp hemp seeds • 2 cups coconut yogurt

• ½ lemon, zested • 3 mint sprigs, chopped • Sugar-free maple syrup to taste

1. In serving glasses, add half of coconut yogurt, cranberries, lemon zest, mint, hemp seeds, and drizzle with maple syrup.

2. Repeat a second layer.

3. Serve with maple syrup.

• Calories: 98

• Fat: 7.8g • Carb: 3.1g • Protein: 4.7g

10 minute prep time Cook time: 10 minutes Servings: 2

• 3 ounces cream cheese • 1 tsp. of ground cinnamon • 1 tbsp. of honey • 1 tsp. of ground cardamom • 1 tsp. of butter • 2 eggs, beaten

1. In a bowl, whisk the eggs finely.

2. Beat the cream cheese in a different bowl until it becomes soft.

3. Add the egg mixture to the softened cream cheese and mix well until there are no lumps left.

4. Add cinnamon, cardamom, and honey to it. Make a thorough mixture. The batter would be runnier than pancake batter.

5. In a pan, add the butter and heat over medium heat.

6. Add the batter using a scooper; that way, all the crepes would be the same size.

7. Fry them golden brown on both sides.

8. Repeat the process with the rest of the batter.

9. Drizzle some honey on top and enjoy.

• Calories: 241

• Fat: 19.8g • Carb: 2.6g • Protein: 10.6g

10 minute prep time Cook time: 12 minutes 4 people

• 1 cup almonds, blanched • 1/3 cup cashew nuts • 2 tbsp coconut oil • Salt as needed • ½ tsp cinnamon

1. Preheat your oven to 350 °F.

2. Bake almonds and cashews for 12 minutes.

3. Let them cool.

4. Transfer to a food processor and add remaining ingredients.

5. Add oil and keep blending until smooth.

6. Serve and enjoy!

• Calories: 278

• Fat: 34g • Carb: 4.6g • Protein: 22g

10 minute prep time Minutes to prepare: 0 6 people

• 1 small package sugar-free cherry gelatin • 1 pie crust, 9-inch size (You can use the recipe "Pie Crust" from this book)

• 8 oz light cream cheese

• 12 oz whipped topping • 20 oz cherry pie filling

1. Prepare the cherry gelatin as per the given instructions on the packet.

2. Pour the mixture in an 8x8 inch pan and refrigerate until set.

3. Soften the cream cheese at room temperature.

4. Place the 9-inch pie crust in a pie pan and bake it until golden brown.

5. Vigorously, beat the cream cheese in a mixer until fluffy and fold in whipped topping.

6. Dice the gelatin into cubes and add them to the cream cheese mixture.

7. Mix gently then add this mixture to the baking pie shell.

8. Top the cream cheese filling with cherry pie filling.

9. Refrigerate for 3 hours then slice to serve.

• Calories: 128

• Fat: 14g • Carb: 4.0g • Protein: 8.1g

10 minute prep time Cook time: 10 minutes Servings: 10

• ½ cup coconut flour • 1 cup blueberries • 2 eggs • ½ cup heavy cream • ½ cup butter • ½ cup almond flour • A pinch of salt • 5 tbsp stevia • 2 tsp vanilla extract • 2 tsp baking powder

1. In a bowl, mix coconut flour and almond flour, salt, baking powder, blueberries, and stir well.

2. In another bowl, mix butter, heavy cream, vanilla extract, stevia, eggs, and stir well.

3. Combine the 2 mixtures and stir until you get a dough.

4. Shape 10 triangles from mixture and place on a lined baking sheet.

5. Place in an oven at 350F and bake for 10 minutes.

6. Serve.

• Calories: 199

• Fat: 16g • Carbs: 4.6g • Protein: 4g

Prep time: 10 minutes + Chilling Cook time: 10 minutes

6 people

• 12 fresh raspberries • 2 cups coconut cream • ½ tbsp powdered gelatin • ¼ tsp vanilla extract • 1tsp turmeric • 1 tbsp Erythritol • 1 tbsp chopped toasted pecans

1. Combine gelatin and ½ tsp water and allow sitting to dissolve.

2. Pour coconut cream, vanilla extract, turmeric, and erythritol into a saucepan and bring to a boil; simmer for 2 minutes. Turn the heat off. Stir in gelatin.

3. Pour into 6 glasses, cover with a plastic wrap, and refrigerate for 2 hours.

4. Top with pecans and raspberries and serve.

• Calories: 218

• Fat: 22g • Carb: 3g • Protein: 4.1g

5 minutes to prepare 5 minutes to prepare 4 people

• 2 tbsp coconut oil • ½ tsp vanilla extract • ½ tsp pumpkin pie spice • 1 tbsp granulated Erythritol • 2 cups unsweetened coconut flakes • 1/8 tsp salt

1. Preheat oven to 350 degrees Fahrenheit (180 degrees Celsius).

2. Melt the coconut oil in the microwave.

3. Add pumpkin pie spice, vanilla extract, and granulated erythritol to coconut oil and mix well.

4. In a bowl, place the coconut flakes.

5. Pour coconut oil mixture over them and toss to coat.

6. Spread out on a single layer on a cookie sheet and sprinkle with salt.

7. Bake until crispy, about 5 minutes.

• Calories: 327

• Fat: 30.4g • Carbs: 4.6g • Protein: 2.8g

10 minute prep time 20-minute cook time Servings: 1 • 2 eggs • 2 tbsp parmesan cheese • 1 tbsp psyllium husk powder

• ½ tsp Italian seasoning • Salt to taste • 2 tsp frying oil • 1 ½ ounce mozzarella cheese • 3 tbsp tomato sauce • 1 tbsp chopped basil

1. In a blender, place the parmesan, psyllium husk powder, Italian seasoning, salt, and two eggs and blend.

2. Heat a large frying pan. Add the oil.

3. Add the mixture to the pan in a large circular shape.

4. Flip once the underside is browning and then remove from the pan.

5. Spoon the tomato sauce onto the pizza crust and spread.

6. Add the cheese and spread over the top of the pizza.

7. Place the pizza into the oven – it is done once the cheese is melted.

8. Top the pizza with basil.

• There are 458 calories in this recipe.

35 grams of fat, 3.5 grams of carbohydrates, and 22 grams of protein

10 minute prep time 25 minutes to prepare 10 servings • 4 cup fresh cranberries • 12 cup water • 2 whole cinnamon sticks • 6 whole cloves • 2 tbsp fresh lemon juice • 12 cup fresh orange juice

1. Bring the cranberries, water, cinnamon sticks, and cloves to a boil in a large saucepan over high heat.

2. Reduce the heat to low and continue to cook for 15-20 minutes, covered.

3. Turn off the stovetop.

4. Pour the tea into a colander lined with cheesecloth.

5. Put the tea back in the pot.

6. Stir in the remaining ingredients.

7. Simmer for approximately 4-5 minutes over medium-low heat, or until the pan is thoroughly heated.

8. Warm up the dish before serving.

• There are 88 calories in a single serving of this dish.

• 0.4 g fat; 2.6 g carbohydrates; 1.9 g protein

5 minutes to prepare 12 minute time to cook 8 tbsp butter • 12 tbsp coconut flour • 1 1/3 cup almond flour • 12 tbsp water

1. In a food processor, combine all of the ingredients until a dough-like consistency is achieved.

2. Fill a pie pan halfway with the mixture.

3. Bake for 14 minutes at 350°F for the prebaked crust.

• There are 65 calories in this recipe.

• 5.4 grams of fat • 2.9 grams of carbohydrates • 1.7 grams of protein

3 hr. 10 min. prep time (with freezing) Minutes to prepare: 0

6 people

• 4 eggs, yolks and whites separated • 14 teaspoon cream of tartar • 12 cup Swerve • 1 teaspoon vanilla essence

1. Combine the egg whites, cream of tartar, and swerve in a mixing bowl. Make a good stir.

2. In a separate bowl, mix together the cream and the vanilla extract.

3. Gently whisk together the 2 ingredients.

4. Whisk egg yolks in a separate dish, then fold in two egg whites.

5. Gently stir the mixture, then place it into a freezer-safe container and freeze for 3 hours before serving.

• 232 kcal

• 23.3 grams of fat; 4.8 grams of carbohydrates; 5.1 grams of protein

45-minute prep time 15-minute time to cook 60 portions

Ingredients

• 12 cup cubed butter plus 1 tsp for greasing • 12 cup whipping cream • 1 cup toasted chopped nuts • 1 tsp vanilla extract • 1 cup powdered sugar

Instructions

In a saucepan, melt the butter and cream. Bring the mixture to a boil while continually stirring it. Cook until a soft ball stage has been achieved.

2. Turn off the heat and stir in the vanilla extract.

3. Allow 30 minutes for cooling.

4. Using a fork, begin to thicken the fudge. Gradually incorporate the powdered sweetener until smooth.

5. Finally, stir in the nuts.

6. Put the fudge on a prepared baking sheet and spread it out evenly.

7. Refrigerate after covering with foil.

8. Cut the foil into squares and remove it from the pan.

Facts on Nutrition (Per Serving)

• 69 calories per serving • 9 grams of fat • 4 grams of carbohydrates • 2 grams of protein

5 minutes to prepare 10 minutes to prepare 2 black tea bags • 1 cup water • 1 entire allspice stick • 1 cinnamon stick

• 2 tablespoons Swerve • 1 cup unsweetened apple juice

1. Bring water, allspice, and the cinnamon stick to a boil in a small saucepan.

2. Cover and remove the tea bags from the heat as soon as possible.

3. Allow 2 minutes for brewing.

4. Discard the allspice berries, cinnamon stick, and tea bags.

5. Cook for 3-5 minutes, or until apple juice and honey are thoroughly heated.

6. Pour the tea into glasses and add honey to taste.

7. Warm up the dish before serving.

• There are 125 calories in this recipe.

• 0.2 g fat; 1.4 g carbohydrate; 0.9 g protein

Marshmallows

10 minute prep time 3 minutes for cooking 6 people

• 2 tbsp gelatin • 12 scoops Stevia • 12 cup cold water • 12 cup hot water • 2 tsp vanilla extract

1. Mix gelatin and cold water in a mixing basin.

2. Combine all of the ingredients in a mixing bowl and let aside for 5 minutes to allow the flavors to meld.

3. In a saucepan, heat the water.

4. Stir in the erythritol and the stevia.

5. Combine the gelatin mixture with it. Mix in the vanilla extract until it is well combined.

6. Using a hand mixer, combine all of the ingredients and pour into a baking dish.

7. Refrigerate for a few hours or overnight to allow the flavors to meld.

8. Serve immediately after cutting.

• 140 Calories

2 g fat, 2 g carbohydrate, 4 g protein

5 minutes to prepare 20 minutes to prepare 6 servings • 1 star anise • 12 whole cloves • 7 whole allspices • 2 cinnamon sticks • 7 entire white peppercorns

2 tbsp black tea leaves • 4 cups milk • 6 tsp Swerve

1. Bring all ingredients to a boil in a saucepan, except the milk and sweetener.

2. Remove from the heat and steep for 20 minutes, covered.

3. Return to a boil by adding the milk.

4. Remove from the heat and steep for 5 minutes, covered.

5. Pour the tea into serving glasses and add sugar to taste.

6. Warm up the dish before serving.

• There are 104 calories in this recipe.

• 4.8 g fat; 3.3 g carbohydrate; 4.9 g protein

5 minutes to prepare 20-minute cook time 14 portions

• 12 cup pumpkin seeds, 12 cup sunflower seeds, 12 cup coarsely chopped almonds, 14 cup unsweetened shredded coconut, 14 cup melted coconut oil, 4 tbsp no sugar added almond butter, 1 tsp vanilla essence, 2 tsp crushed cinnamon, 1/8 tsp salt, 3 tbsp granular swerve

1. Preheat oven to 350 degrees Fahrenheit (180 degrees Celsius).

2. Pulse almonds and seeds in a food processor until they're somewhat broken up.

3. Pulse in the rest of the ingredients until well combined.

4. Pour mixture into a silicone baking dish that measures 8 by 8 inches.

5. Preheat the oven to 200°F and bake for 20 minutes.

6. Allow to cool before slicing.

• There are 165 calories in a single serving of this dish.

• 14.4 g fat • 5.7 g carbohydrate • 5.1 g protein• There are 458 calories in this recipe.

35 grams of fat, 3.5 grams of carbohydrates, and 22 grams of protein

10 minute prep time 25 minutes to prepare 10 servings • 4 cup fresh cranberries • 12 cup water • 2 whole cinnamon sticks • 6 whole cloves • 2 tbsp fresh lemon juice • 12 cup fresh orange juice

1. Bring the cranberries, water, cinnamon sticks, and cloves to a boil in a large saucepan over high heat.

2. Reduce the heat to low and continue to cook for 15-20 minutes, covered.

3. Turn off the stovetop.

4. Pour the tea into a colander lined with cheesecloth.

5. Put the tea back in the pot.

6. Stir in the remaining ingredients.

7. Simmer for approximately 4-5 minutes over medium-low heat, or until the pan is thoroughly heated.

8. Warm up the dish before serving.

• There are 88 calories in a single serving of this dish.

• 0.4 g fat; 2.6 g carbohydrates; 1.9 g protein

5 minutes to prepare 12 minute time to cook 8 tbsp butter • 12 tbsp coconut flour • 1 1/3 cup almond flour • 12 tbsp water

1. In a food processor, combine all of the ingredients until a dough-like consistency is achieved.

2. Fill a pie pan halfway with the mixture.

3. Bake for 14 minutes at 350°F for the prebaked crust.

• There are 65 calories in this recipe.

• 5.4 grams of fat • 2.9 grams of carbohydrates • 1.7 grams of protein

3 hr. 10 min. prep time (with freezing) Minutes to prepare: 0

6 people

• 4 eggs, yolks and whites separated • 14 teaspoon cream of tartar • 12 cup Swerve • 1 teaspoon vanilla essence

1. Combine the egg whites, cream of tartar, and swerve in a mixing bowl. Make a good stir.

2. In a separate bowl, mix together the cream and the vanilla extract.

3. Gently whisk together the 2 ingredients.

4. Whisk egg yolks in a separate dish, then fold in two egg whites.

5. Gently stir the mixture, then place it into a freezer-safe container and freeze for 3 hours before serving.

• 232 kcal

• 23.3 grams of fat; 4.8 grams of carbohydrates; 5.1 grams of protein

45-minute prep time 15-minute time to cook 60 portions

Ingredients

• 12 cup cubed butter plus 1 tsp for greasing • 12 cup whipping cream • 1 cup toasted chopped nuts • 1 tsp vanilla extract • 1 cup powdered sugar

Instructions

In a saucepan, melt the butter and cream. Bring the mixture to a boil while continually stirring it. Cook until a soft ball stage has been achieved.

2. Turn off the heat and stir in the vanilla extract.

3. Allow 30 minutes for cooling.

4. Using a fork, begin to thicken the fudge. Gradually incorporate the powdered sweetener until smooth.

5. Finally, stir in the nuts.

6. Put the fudge on a prepared baking sheet and spread it out evenly.

7. Refrigerate after covering with foil.

8. Cut the foil into squares and remove it from the pan.

Facts on Nutrition (Per Serving)

• 69 calories per serving • 9 grams of fat • 4 grams of carbohydrates • 2 grams of protein

5 minutes to prepare 10 minutes to prepare 2 black tea bags • 1 cup water • 1 entire allspice stick • 1 cinnamon stick

• 2 tablespoons Swerve • 1 cup unsweetened apple juice

1. Bring water, allspice, and the cinnamon stick to a boil in a small saucepan.

2. Cover and remove the tea bags from the heat as soon as possible.

3. Allow 2 minutes for brewing.

4. Discard the allspice berries, cinnamon stick, and tea bags.

5. Cook for 3-5 minutes, or until apple juice and honey are thoroughly heated.

6. Pour the tea into glasses and add honey to taste.

7. Warm up the dish before serving.

• There are 125 calories in this recipe.

• 0.2 g fat; 1.4 g carbohydrate; 0.9 g protein

Marshmallows

10 minute prep time 3 minutes for cooking 6 people

• 2 tbsp gelatin • 12 scoops Stevia • 12 cup cold water • 12 cup hot water • 2 tsp vanilla extract

1. Mix gelatin and cold water in a mixing basin.

2. Combine all of the ingredients in a mixing bowl and let aside for 5 minutes to allow the flavors to meld.

3. In a saucepan, heat the water.

4. Stir in the erythritol and the stevia.

5. Combine the gelatin mixture with it. Mix in the vanilla extract until it is well combined.

6. Using a hand mixer, combine all of the ingredients and pour into a baking dish.

7. Refrigerate for a few hours or overnight to allow the flavors to meld.

8. Serve immediately after cutting.

• 140 Calories

2 g fat, 2 g carbohydrate, 4 g protein

5 minutes to prepare 20 minutes to prepare 6 servings • 1 star anise • 12 whole cloves • 7 whole allspices • 2 cinnamon sticks • 7 entire white peppercorns

2 tbsp black tea leaves • 4 cups milk • 6 tsp Swerve

1. Bring all ingredients to a boil in a saucepan, except the milk and sweetener.

2. Remove from the heat and steep for 20 minutes, covered.

3. Return to a boil by adding the milk.

4. Remove from the heat and steep for 5 minutes, covered.

5. Pour the tea into serving glasses and add sugar to taste.

6. Warm up the dish before serving.

• There are 104 calories in this recipe.

• 4.8 g fat; 3.3 g carbohydrate; 4.9 g protein

5 minutes to prepare 20-minute cook time 14 portions

• 12 cup pumpkin seeds, 12 cup sunflower seeds, 12 cup coarsely chopped almonds, 14 cup unsweetened shredded coconut, 14 cup melted coconut oil, 4 tbsp no sugar added almond butter, 1 tsp vanilla essence, 2 tsp crushed cinnamon, 1/8 tsp salt, 3 tbsp granular swerve

1. Preheat oven to 350 degrees Fahrenheit (180 degrees Celsius).

2. Pulse almonds and seeds in a food processor until they're somewhat broken up.

3. Pulse in the rest of the ingredients until well combined.

4. Pour mixture into a silicone baking dish that measures 8 by 8 inches.

5. Preheat the oven to 200°F and bake for 20 minutes.

6. Allow to cool before slicing.

• There are 165 calories in a single serving of this dish.

• 14.4 g fat • 5.7 g carbohydrate • 5.1 g protein• There are 458 calories in this recipe.

35 grams of fat, 3.5 grams of carbohydrates, and 22 grams of protein

10 minute prep time 25 minutes to prepare 10 servings • 4 cup fresh cranberries • 12 cup water • 2 whole cinnamon sticks • 6 whole cloves • 2 tbsp fresh lemon juice • 12 cup fresh orange juice

1. Bring the cranberries, water, cinnamon sticks, and cloves to a boil in a large saucepan over high heat.

2. Reduce the heat to low and continue to cook for 15-20 minutes, covered.

3. Turn off the stovetop.

4. Pour the tea into a colander lined with cheesecloth.

5. Put the tea back in the pot.

6. Stir in the remaining ingredients.

7. Simmer for approximately 4-5 minutes over medium-low heat, or until the pan is thoroughly heated.

8. Warm up the dish before serving.

• There are 88 calories in a single serving of this dish.

• 0.4 g fat; 2.6 g carbohydrates; 1.9 g protein

5 minutes to prepare 12 minute time to cook 8 tbsp butter • 12 tbsp coconut flour • 1 1/3 cup almond flour • 12 tbsp water

1. In a food processor, combine all of the ingredients until a dough-like consistency is achieved.

2. Fill a pie pan halfway with the mixture.

3. Bake for 14 minutes at 350°F for the prebaked crust.

• There are 65 calories in this recipe.

• 5.4 grams of fat • 2.9 grams of carbohydrates • 1.7 grams of protein

3 hr. 10 min. prep time (with freezing) Minutes to prepare: 0

6 people

• 4 eggs, yolks and whites separated • 14 teaspoon cream of tartar • 12 cup Swerve • 1 teaspoon vanilla essence

1. Combine the egg whites, cream of tartar, and swerve in a mixing bowl. Make a good stir.

2. In a separate bowl, mix together the cream and the vanilla extract.

3. Gently whisk together the 2 ingredients.

4. Whisk egg yolks in a separate dish, then fold in two egg whites.

5. Gently stir the mixture, then place it into a freezer-safe container and freeze for 3 hours before serving.

• 232 kcal

• 23.3 grams of fat; 4.8 grams of carbohydrates; 5.1 grams of protein

45-minute prep time 15-minute time to cook 60 portions

Ingredients

• 12 cup cubed butter plus 1 tsp for greasing • 12 cup whipping cream • 1 cup toasted chopped nuts • 1 tsp vanilla extract • 1 cup powdered sugar

Instructions

In a saucepan, melt the butter and cream. Bring the mixture to a boil while continually stirring it. Cook until a soft ball stage has been achieved.

2. Turn off the heat and stir in the vanilla extract.

3. Allow 30 minutes for cooling.

4. Using a fork, begin to thicken the fudge. Gradually incorporate the powdered sweetener until smooth.

5. Finally, stir in the nuts.

6. Put the fudge on a prepared baking sheet and spread it out evenly.

7. Refrigerate after covering with foil.

8. Cut the foil into squares and remove it from the pan.

Facts on Nutrition (Per Serving)

• 69 calories per serving • 9 grams of fat • 4 grams of carbohydrates • 2 grams of protein

5 minutes to prepare 10 minutes to prepare 2 black tea bags • 1 cup water • 1 entire allspice stick • 1 cinnamon stick

• 2 tablespoons Swerve • 1 cup unsweetened apple juice

1. Bring water, allspice, and the cinnamon stick to a boil in a small saucepan.

2. Cover and remove the tea bags from the heat as soon as possible.

3. Allow 2 minutes for brewing.

4. Discard the allspice berries, cinnamon stick, and tea bags.

5. Cook for 3-5 minutes, or until apple juice and honey are thoroughly heated.

6. Pour the tea into glasses and add honey to taste.

7. Warm up the dish before serving.

• There are 125 calories in this recipe.

• 0.2 g fat; 1.4 g carbohydrate; 0.9 g protein

Marshmallows

10 minute prep time 3 minutes for cooking 6 people

• 2 tbsp gelatin • 12 scoops Stevia • 12 cup cold water • 12 cup hot water • 2 tsp vanilla extract

1. Mix gelatin and cold water in a mixing basin.

2. Combine all of the ingredients in a mixing bowl and let aside for 5 minutes to allow the flavors to meld.

3. In a saucepan, heat the water.

4. Stir in the erythritol and the stevia.

5. Combine the gelatin mixture with it. Mix in the vanilla extract until it is well combined.

6. Using a hand mixer, combine all of the ingredients and pour into a baking dish.

7. Refrigerate for a few hours or overnight to allow the flavors to meld.

8. Serve immediately after cutting.

• 140 Calories

2 g fat, 2 g carbohydrate, 4 g protein

5 minutes to prepare 20 minutes to prepare 6 servings • 1 star anise • 12 whole cloves • 7 whole allspices • 2 cinnamon sticks • 7 entire white peppercorns

2 tbsp black tea leaves • 4 cups milk • 6 tsp Swerve

1. Bring all ingredients to a boil in a saucepan, except the milk and sweetener.

2. Remove from the heat and steep for 20 minutes, covered.

3. Return to a boil by adding the milk.

4. Remove from the heat and steep for 5 minutes, covered.

5. Pour the tea into serving glasses and add sugar to taste.

6. Warm up the dish before serving.

• There are 104 calories in this recipe.

• 4.8 g fat; 3.3 g carbohydrate; 4.9 g protein

5 minutes to prepare 20-minute cook time 14 portions

• 12 cup pumpkin seeds, 12 cup sunflower seeds, 12 cup coarsely chopped almonds, 14 cup unsweetened shredded coconut, 14 cup melted coconut oil, 4 tbsp no sugar added almond butter, 1 tsp vanilla essence, 2 tsp crushed cinnamon, 1/8 tsp salt, 3 tbsp granular swerve

1. Preheat oven to 350 degrees Fahrenheit (180 degrees Celsius).

2. Pulse almonds and seeds in a food processor until they're somewhat broken up.

3. Pulse in the rest of the ingredients until well combined.

4. Pour mixture into a silicone baking dish that measures 8 by 8 inches.

5. Preheat the oven to 200°F and bake for 20 minutes.

6. Allow to cool before slicing.

• There are 165 calories in a single serving of this dish.

• 14.4 g fat • 5.7 g carbohydrate • 5.1 g protein• There are 458 calories in this recipe.

35 grams of fat, 3.5 grams of carbohydrates, and 22 grams of protein

10 minute prep time 25 minutes to prepare 10 servings • 4 cup fresh cranberries • 12 cup water • 2 whole cinnamon sticks • 6 whole cloves • 2 tbsp fresh lemon juice • 12 cup fresh orange juice

1. Bring the cranberries, water, cinnamon sticks, and cloves to a boil in a large saucepan over high heat.

2. Reduce the heat to low and continue to cook for 15-20 minutes, covered.

3. Turn off the stovetop.

4. Pour the tea into a colander lined with cheesecloth.

5. Put the tea back in the pot.

6. Stir in the remaining ingredients.

7. Simmer for approximately 4-5 minutes over medium-low heat, or until the pan is thoroughly heated.

8. Warm up the dish before serving.

• There are 88 calories in a single serving of this dish.

• 0.4 g fat; 2.6 g carbohydrates; 1.9 g protein

5 minutes to prepare 12 minute time to cook 8 tbsp butter • 12 tbsp coconut flour • 1 1/3 cup almond flour • 12 tbsp water

1. In a food processor, combine all of the ingredients until a dough-like consistency is achieved.

2. Fill a pie pan halfway with the mixture.

3. Bake for 14 minutes at 350°F for the prebaked crust.

• There are 65 calories in this recipe.

• 5.4 grams of fat • 2.9 grams of carbohydrates • 1.7 grams of protein

3 hr. 10 min. prep time (with freezing) Minutes to prepare: 0

6 people

• 4 eggs, yolks and whites separated • 14 teaspoon cream of tartar • 12 cup Swerve • 1 teaspoon vanilla essence

1. Combine the egg whites, cream of tartar, and swerve in a mixing bowl. Make a good stir.

2. In a separate bowl, mix together the cream and the vanilla extract.

3. Gently whisk together the 2 ingredients.

4. Whisk egg yolks in a separate dish, then fold in two egg whites.

5. Gently stir the mixture, then place it into a freezer-safe container and freeze for 3 hours before serving.

• 232 kcal

• 23.3 grams of fat; 4.8 grams of carbohydrates; 5.1 grams of protein

45-minute prep time 15-minute time to cook 60 portions

Ingredients

• 12 cup cubed butter plus 1 tsp for greasing • 12 cup whipping cream • 1 cup toasted chopped nuts • 1 tsp vanilla extract • 1 cup powdered sugar

Instructions

In a saucepan, melt the butter and cream. Bring the mixture to a boil while continually stirring it. Cook until a soft ball stage has been achieved.

2. Turn off the heat and stir in the vanilla extract.

3. Allow 30 minutes for cooling.

4. Using a fork, begin to thicken the fudge. Gradually incorporate the powdered sweetener until smooth.

5. Finally, stir in the nuts.

6. Put the fudge on a prepared baking sheet and spread it out evenly.

7. Refrigerate after covering with foil.

8. Cut the foil into squares and remove it from the pan.

Facts on Nutrition (Per Serving)

• 69 calories per serving • 9 grams of fat • 4 grams of carbohydrates • 2 grams of protein

5 minutes to prepare 10 minutes to prepare 2 black tea bags • 1 cup water • 1 entire allspice stick • 1 cinnamon stick

• 2 tablespoons Swerve • 1 cup unsweetened apple juice

1. Bring water, allspice, and the cinnamon stick to a boil in a small saucepan.

2. Cover and remove the tea bags from the heat as soon as possible.

3. Allow 2 minutes for brewing.

4. Discard the allspice berries, cinnamon stick, and tea bags.

5. Cook for 3-5 minutes, or until apple juice and honey are thoroughly heated.

6. Pour the tea into glasses and add honey to taste.

7. Warm up the dish before serving.

• There are 125 calories in this recipe.

• 0.2 g fat; 1.4 g carbohydrate; 0.9 g protein

Chapter Ten

Marshmallows

Marshmallows

10 minute prep time 3 minutes for cooking 6 people

• 2 tbsp gelatin • 12 scoops Stevia • 12 cup cold water • 12 cup hot water • 2 tsp vanilla extract

1. Mix gelatin and cold water in a mixing basin.

2. Combine all of the ingredients in a mixing bowl and let aside for 5 minutes to allow the flavors to meld.

3. In a saucepan, heat the water.

4. Stir in the erythritol and the stevia.

5. Combine the gelatin mixture with it. Mix in the vanilla extract until it is well combined.

6. Using a hand mixer, combine all of the ingredients and pour into a baking dish.

7. Refrigerate for a few hours or overnight to allow the flavors to meld.

8. Serve immediately after cutting.

• 140 Calories

2 g fat, 2 g carbohydrate, 4 g protein

5 minutes to prepare 20 minutes to prepare 6 servings • 1 star anise • 12 whole cloves • 7 whole allspices • 2 cinnamon sticks • 7 entire white peppercorns

2 tbsp black tea leaves • 4 cups milk • 6 tsp Swerve

1. Bring all ingredients to a boil in a saucepan, except the milk and sweetener.

2. Remove from the heat and steep for 20 minutes, covered.

3. Return to a boil by adding the milk.

4. Remove from the heat and steep for 5 minutes, covered.

5. Pour the tea into serving glasses and add sugar to taste.

6. Warm up the dish before serving.

• There are 104 calories in this recipe.

• 4.8 g fat; 3.3 g carbohydrate; 4.9 g protein

5 minutes to prepare 20-minute cook time 14 portions

• 12 cup pumpkin seeds, 12 cup sunflower seeds, 12 cup coarsely chopped almonds, 14 cup unsweetened shredded coconut, 14 cup melted coconut oil, 4 tbsp no sugar added almond butter, 1 tsp vanilla essence, 2 tsp crushed cinnamon, 1/8 tsp salt, 3 tbsp granular swerve

1. Preheat oven to 350 degrees Fahrenheit (180 degrees Celsius).

2. Pulse almonds and seeds in a food processor until they're somewhat broken up.

3. Pulse in the rest of the ingredients until well combined.

4. Pour mixture into a silicone baking dish that measures 8 by 8 inches.

5. Preheat the oven to 200°F and bake for 20 minutes.

6. Allow to cool before slicing.

• There are 165 calories in a single serving of this dish.

• 14.4 g fat • 5.7 g carbohydrate • 5.1 g protein

CPSIA information can be obtained
at www.ICGtesting.com
Printed in the USA
BVHW092118200322
631968BV00014B/706